# Clinical Electrophysiology
# Review

**George J. Klein, M.D.**
*Professor of Medicine*
*Head, Division of Cardiology*
*University of Western Ontario*
*London, Ontario, Canada*

**Eric N. Prystowsky, M.D.**
*Northside Cardiology, PC*
*Indianapolis, Indiana*
*Consulting Professor of Medicine*
*Duke University Medical Center*
*Durham, North Carolina*

**McGRAW-IIILL**
**Health Professions Division**

New York  St. Louis  San Francisco  Auckland  Bogotá
Caracas  Lisbon  London  Madrid  Mexico City  Milan  Montreal
New Delhi  San Juan  Singapore  Sydney  Tokyo  Toronto

**McGraw-Hill**

*A Division of The McGraw-Hill Companies*

1 2 3 4 5 6 7 8 9 0   MALMAL   9 8 7 6

ISBN 0-07-035169-4

This book was set in Times Roman by Bi-Comp, Inc.
The editors were Joe Hefta and Peter McCurdy; the production supervisor was Clare Stanley; the cover designer was Ed Schultheis.
Malloy Lithographics was printer and binder.
The project was managed by Spectrum Publisher Services.

This book is printed on acid-free paper.


**Library of Congress Cataloging-in-Publication Data**

Klein, George J.
    Clinical electrophysiology review / George J. Klein, Eric N. Prystowsky.
       p.  cm.
    Includes bibliographical references and index.
    ISBN 0-07-035169-4
    1. Electrocardiography—Case studies.  2. Arrhythmia—Diagnosis—Case studies.  I. Prystowsky, Eric N.  II. Title.
    [DNLM: 1. Arrhythmia—diagnosis—case studies.  2. Arrhythmia—examination questions.  3. Electrocardiography—examination questions.  4. Electrophysiology—examination questions.  WG 330 K64c 1996]
RC683.5.E5K53  1996
616.1'2807547'076  dc20
DNLM/DLC
for Library of Congress                        96-43397
                                              CIP

# Clinical Electrophysiology
# Review

# NOTICE

# Contents

# *Preface*

We of the "old school" remember training when clinical electrophysiology was in its infancy and little was known of the mechanism of the commonly encountered arrhythmias. Every case was a puzzle that provoked scholarly discussion, fanciful hypotheses, and plans for future research. Decades later, we have entered into the exciting era of interventional electrophysiology where we walk into the laboratory with the expectation that we will not only unravel the mechanism of the arrhythmia but *cure* the patient before the catheters are removed! A disturbing corollary of this progress has been a deemphasis on the fundamentals of the diagnostic study and a focus on an expedient ablation procedure. Many trainees show little interest in the nuances and subtleties of electrophysiologic diagnosis, an unfortunate trend that will diminish their ability to assess complex problems. We hope that the cases presented in this text will help in a small way to rekindle interest in the gratification of solving an arrhythmia puzzle that ultimately will lead to better care for our patients.

We are indebted to Mrs. Mary Kay Franklin for her outstanding secretarial assistance and to George Moogk and Mrs. Jane E. Gilmore, C.M.T., for their expert artwork.

This book is dedicated to our students who have learned from us, taught us, and inspired us with their enthusiasm.

George J. Klein
Eric N. Prystowsky

# Clinical Electrophysiology
# Review

# Chapter 1

# Analysis of Complex Electrophysiologic Data

A novice in a busy electrophysiology (EP) laboratory will generally learn to recognize the common arrhythmias in a relatively short time. It requires considerably more seasoning to recognize the variants and unusual mechanisms, or to "hit the curve ball." It is hoped that the following commentary assists in providing structure and focus to the EP study and facilitates analysis of the case studies to follow.

## It Begins with the Electrocardiogram

The electrophysiology study is an extension of the electrocardiogram (ECG) with the addition of intracardiac recording and programmed electrical stimulation. Insightful interpretation of the ECG allows for prospectively considering additional catheters, stimulation sequences, or maneuvers appropriate for the postulated arrhythmia. This limits the diagnostic possibilities and avoids unnecessary steps (Fig. 1–1). The fundamentals of ECG interpretation of an arrhythmia include identification of P waves, determining the atrioventricular (AV) relationship and analyzing the QRS morphology (Table 1–1). For confusing problems, it is useful to create a "written" list of all potential hypotheses and to plan for specific interventions that will test them. As data are accumulated during the EP study, the facts supporting or refuting the hypotheses can be tabulated. The hypotheses can be represented by schematic drawings for complicated scenarios. This method is illustrated at the end of this chapter.

## Less Is Often Not More

There are those gifted, intuitive individuals who leap to the correct diagnosis and apparently bypass all the rational, systematic steps. Most of us, however, are better served by a consistent, methodical approach that does not cut corners. A sample protocol for an unknown tachycardia is shown in Table 1–2. When used routinely, such a protocol will usually result in induction of clinically relevant tachycardia and provide an assessment of the pertinent electrophysiology of the heart. Determining the functional properties of the atria, ventricles, and AV conduction system in an individual elucidates the potential arrhythmia mechanisms and limits the diagnostic possibilities for the observed arrhythmia. For example, it is difficult to imagine AV reentrant tachycardia occurring in the total absence of retrograde conduction. It is also important to display the data channels in a consistent sequence to provide an orderly and familiar framework that facilitates analysis. This point is underscored by the fact that even experienced electrophysiologists require a period of adjustment when looking at data from other laboratories. Of course, other nonconventional recording sites can be added to facilitate diagnosis in selected cases. For example, recording from the left bundle branch can be useful when confirming the diagnosis of bundle branch reentrant tachycardia.

A thorough diagnostic study need not be time consuming and pays dividends both intellectually and clinically. The temptation to ablate an obvious accessory pathway (AP) without study will not be productive if the patient's symptoms are not related to any tachycardia, the patient's tachycardia is not related to the pathway, or the "culprit" AP is a different pathway (Fig. 1–2). The study also provides information regarding other potential rhythm problems that may be unrecognized during the clinical assessment and allows consideration of alternative approaches such as slow pathway ablation in a patient with AV reentrant tachycardia that can only occur with anterograde conduction over the slow AV node pathway. Radiofrequency ablation itself is an important diagnostic tool. Cases

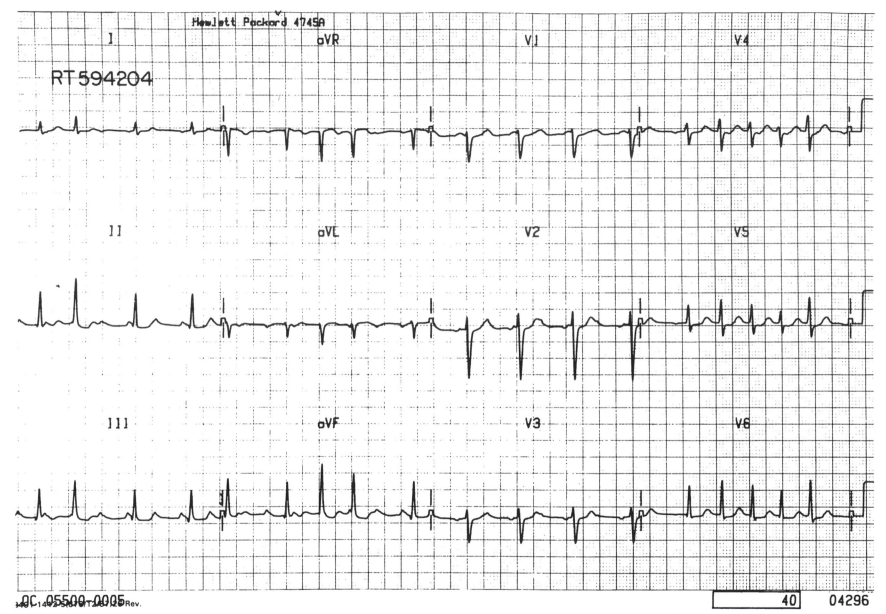

**1–1** Twelve-lead ECG in a patient with palpitations. Inspection of the frontal leads reveals atrial tachycardia with variable AV conduction. The axis of the ectopic P wave (negative in lead I) indicates the diagnosis of "left atrial tachycar-dia." This information provides a focused starting point to plan catheter ablation, if indicated.

involving multiple tachycardia mechanisms can be very confusing. In such situations, at least one of the tachycardia mechanisms is frequently obvious and successful ablation of the tachycardia generally simplifies the diagnosis of the remaining mechanism(s).

## The Key Is Frequently at a Transition

Fishermen have long appreciated that the majority of the fish are caught in a relatively small area of the lake. Similarly, the correct diagnosis may not be apparent from the copious EP records during stable tachycardia. Although the electrograms may have a certain temporal sequence, there is no indication of cause and effect in the sequence of electrograms. Is the atrium driving the ventricle or vice versa? Is the preexcited QRS an active participant in the tachycardia circuit or merely a bystander camouflaging another mechanism? The "hot spots" that frequently yield the answer are the *zones of*

*transition.* The zones include the *onset* of tachycardia, the *termination* of tachycardia, change to an *alternate QRS morphology, irregularities in cycle length,* and *ectopic cycles* (Table 1–3). The onset reveals the conditions necessary to initiate the tachycardia. Does it require block in an AP, critical prolongation of the atrio-His (AH) interval, or conduction delay in the His-Purkinje system? Does a supraventricular tachycardia (SVT) consistently terminate spontaneously with an atrial electrogram? The latter strongly suggests that the tachycardia mechanism obligates AV node conduction. Does a change from normal QRS to bundle branch block alter any of the conduction intervals or tachycardia cycle length, suggesting the bundle branch is a critical component of the tachycardia circuit? Careful attention to the zones of transition is often rewarding as is illustrated.

## Make Something Happen

The EP study provides an opportunity to disturb an arrhythmia with pacing, extrastimuli, autonomic maneuvers, physical maneuvers, and drugs. Single, or multiple, atrial or ventricular extrastimuli are programmed into the cardiac cycle and made progressively more premature to loss of capture. This invariably provides the zone of transition that clarifies the requirement of atrium or ventricle in the mechanism or alters the tachycardia in a manner that clarifies the problem. In other words, "if the tachycardia mechanism is obscure, premature it." We stress the "inverse rule" of EP to our trainees . . . initially introduce premature atrial extrasystoles into a wide QRS tachycardia and ventricular extrasystoles into a narrow QRS tachycardia. Changes in posture cause autonomic adjustments and alter cardiac filling. Agents such as adenosine affect specific tissues and mechanisms, and can be invaluable. Isoproterenol is useful for mimicking states of catecholamine excess or altering specific EP properties to allow induction of tachycardia.

## Expect the Unexpected

It is important to keep an open mind to all the diagnostic possibilities until the correct one has been clearly established. Prematurely accepting what appears to be obvious may result in the psychological

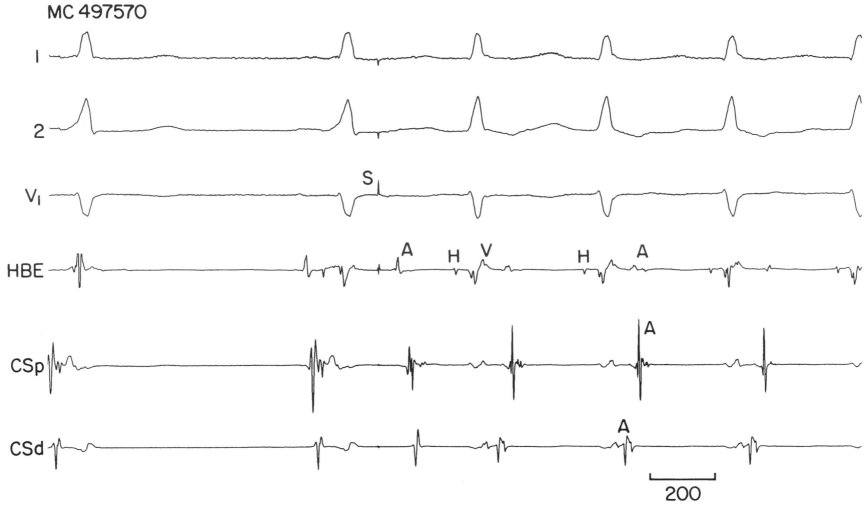

MC 497570

I

2

V₁                                    S

HBE                         A    H   V        H    A

CSp                                              A

CSd                                        A

                                    |———| 200

**1–2**  Tracing from a patient with Wolff-Parkinson-White (WPW) and documented supraventricular tachycardia. The first two cycles are preexcited and a
12-lead ECG suggested a septal pathway conducting anterogradely. Earliest
ventricular activation in sinus rhythm is at the proximal coronary sinus electrode
(CSp) positioned near the orifice of the coronary sinus. An atrial extrastimulus
(S) blocks the pathway and starts supraventricular tachycardia. However, earliest retrograde atrial activity is at the *distal* coronary sinus electrogram. In this
patient, complete mapping revealed that the "culprit" accessory pathway was a
concealed left lateral pathway and the manifest accessory pathway was of no
clinical significance. Ablation of this pathway would have served no purpose. 1,
2, V₁, surface ECG; HBE, His bundle electrogram.

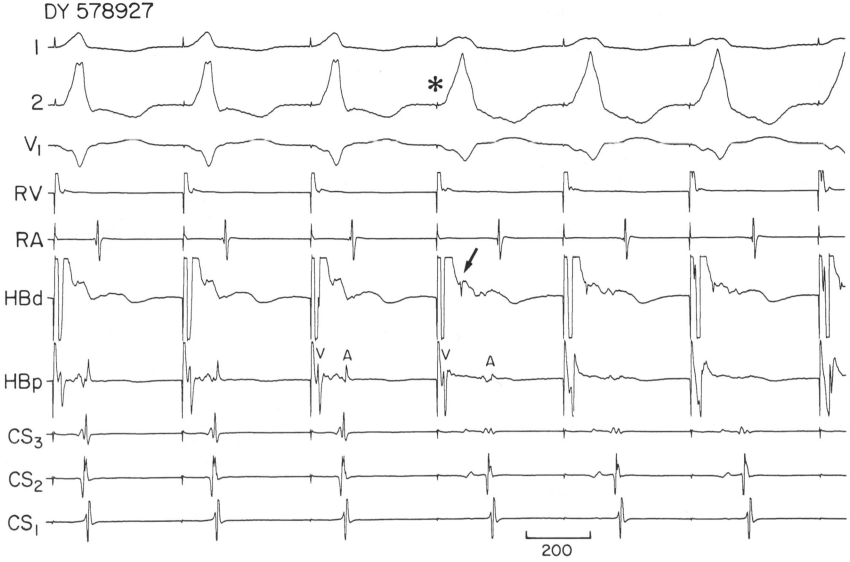

**1–3** Evaluation of retrograde conduction during EP testing. This patient had nondecremental, concentric retrograde atrial conduction and it was unclear whether retrograde conduction was proceeding over the normal AV node or over a concealed accessory pathway. His bundle pacing is achieved (first three cycles) by pacing the distal pole of the His catheter. As the current strength is reduced, His bundle capture is lost and the adjacent RV myocardium is paced. This is indicated by the widening of the QRS (*asterisk*) and the appearance of a retrograde His potential (*arrow*). This clearly indicates that retrograde conduction was proceeding over the AV node since conduction over an anteroseptal AP would not be affected by the loss of His bundle capture. Λ, atrial electrogram; CS, coronary sinus electrograms from proximal (3) to distal (1), respectively; HB, His bundle electrograms from the distal (d) and proximal (p) poles of the catheter; RA, RV, right atrial and ventricular electrograms, respectively; V, ventricular electrogram.

**Table 1–3   Zones of Transition: The Key to the Mechanism**

- The onset of tachycardia
- The termination of tachycardia
- Change to an alternate QRS morphology
- Irregularities in cycle length
- Ectopic cycles

trap of fitting subsequent observations to the expected and may blind a person from performing the required steps. For example, a SVT with simultaneous atrial and ventricular activation immediately suggests AV node reentry but does not rule out atrial tachycardia with a long AV interval or junctional tachycardia with retrograde conduction.

## You Must Have the Tools

An organized approach and strategic plan are only useful with a firm knowledge of physiologic principles and mechanisms. Consider an example where ventricular pacing produces a "central" (concentric) retrograde activation sequence with earliest retrograde atrial activation at the His bundle electrogram. Retrograde conduction time is constant (not rate dependent), and there is no suggestion of anterograde preexcitation. Is retrograde conduction proceeding over the AV node, or is it proceeding over a "concealed" septal AP? Block of retrograde conduction with adenosine favors but does not definitively prove AV node conduction since adenosine may affect some APs. A fundamental physiologic principle can be applied. The ventriculoatrial (VA) conduction will be shortest when pacing at the ventricular site closest to the retrograde pathway. In the case of an anteroseptal AP, pacing the ventricle near the His bundle will provide the shortest VA interval (assuming one does not use sufficient energy to cause His bundle capture). In the case of AV node conduction, pacing near the terminus of the right bundle branch (the RV apex is close to this) will provide the shorter VA interval when pacing at the same rate. This principle is illustrated in Fig. 1–3. Pacing the His bundle directly will result in very early capture of the atrium

near the His bundle. Loss of His bundle capture (by lowering current strength) and remaining capture of myocardium in the region will result in VA prolongation if conduction was proceeding over the AV node but no change in this interval if retrograde conduction was proceeding over an anteroseptal AP. As another example, AV node conduction is rate dependent (decremental) with prolongation of the AH interval after progressively more premature atrial extrastimuli while AP conduction is generally not rate dependent. However, it is important to appreciate that some APs exhibit impressive rate dependence comparable to the AV node, whereas other AV nodes exhibit little or no rate dependence and mimic AP conduction. There is no shortcut to the assimilation of EP principles.

A differential diagnosis of potential entities when a phenomenon is encountered is a fundamental tool to begin the process of hypothesis testing to arrive at the correct diagnosis. Tables 1–4 to 1–10 may be useful in this regard in the analysis of the unknown traces.

## The Electrophysiology Study: An Application of Hypothesis Testing

An orderly EP study is an exercise in establishing a differential diagnosis and systematically gathering evidence to arrive at the correct one. Analysis of an unknown tracing is easier in the context of a real study where one has the advantage of building on information and applying interventions to assist the process. Nonetheless, the exercise of interpreting an unknown trace out of context is an effective learning tool. Review of an unknown EP record is fundamentally the same as reading an ECG with the advantage (and challenge) of the intracardiac recordings. An approach to this analysis is outlined in Table 1–11 and is illustrated in the following examples.

### *Example A*
The patient whose trace is shown in Fig. 1–4 is a young man with recent onset of paroxysmal tachycardia.

The surface leads show the onset of a regular wide QRS rhythm with left bundle branch block pattern. The intracardiac records indicate two tachycardias, clearly of different mechanisms because of

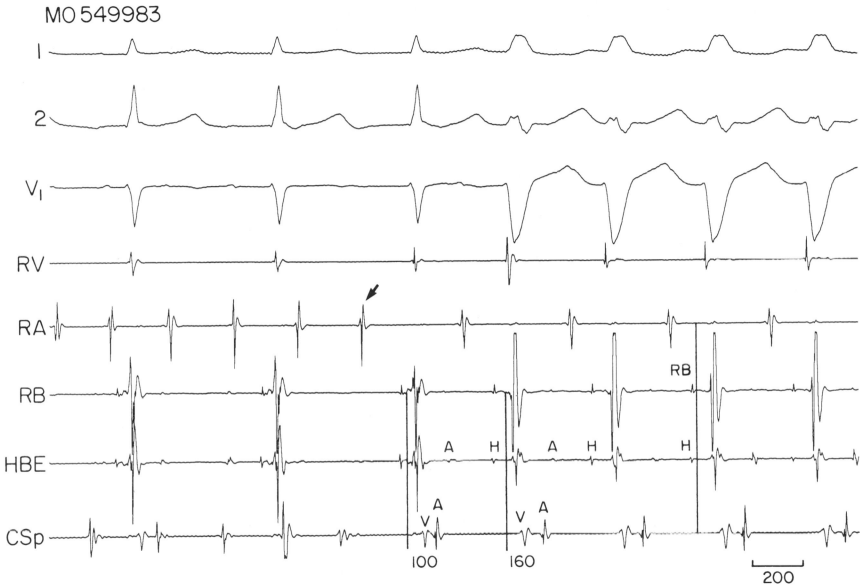

**1-4** Tracing from patient described in example A (see text). H, His bundle electrogram; RB, right bundle branch electrogram.

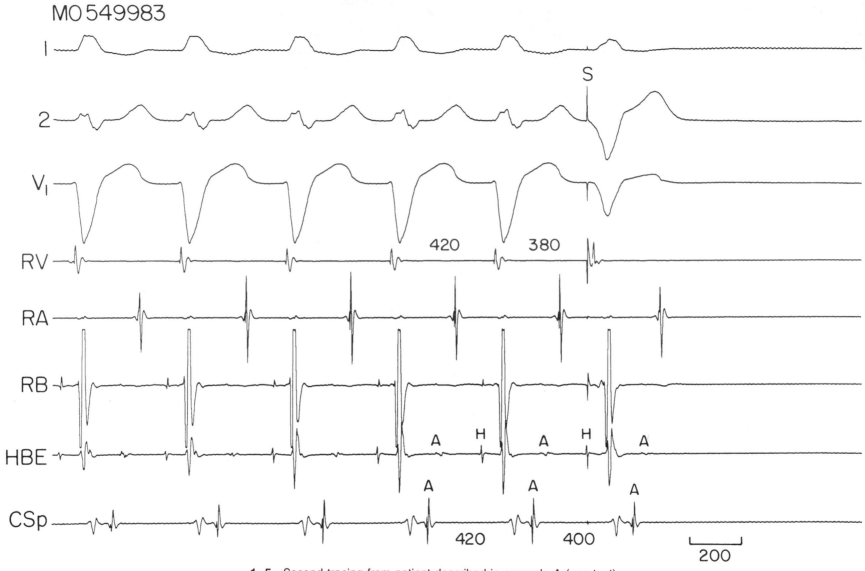

**1–5** Second tracing from patient described in example A (see text).

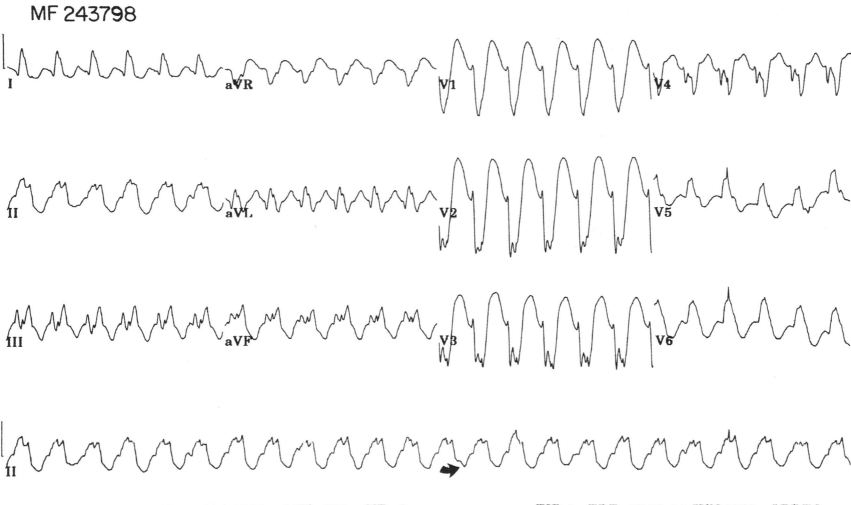

MF 243798

I    aVR    V1    V4

II    aVL    V2    V5

III    aVF    V3    V6

II

mm/s    10mm/mV    150Hz    003A-003A    12SL 250    CID: 3        EID:4    EDT: 15:03 14-JUN-1995    ORDER:

**1-6**    ECG during tachycardia from patient in example B (see text).

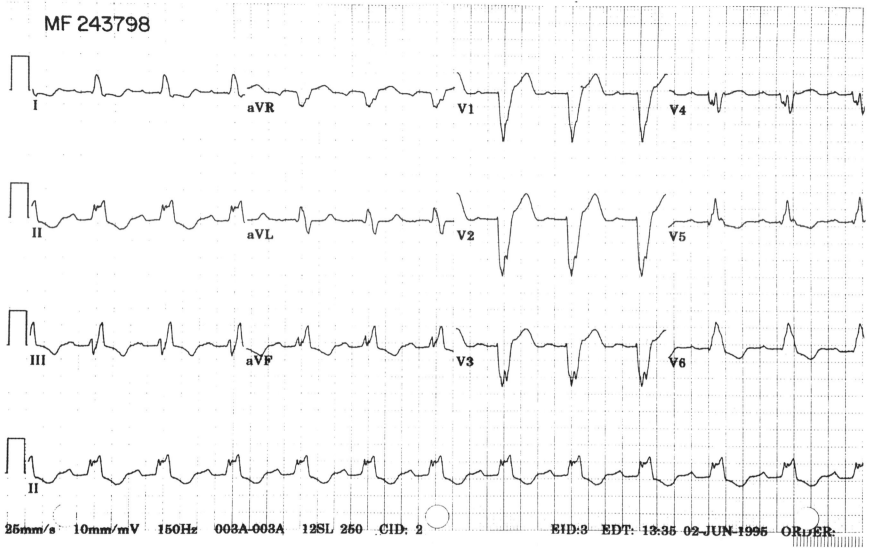

MF 243798

I  aVR  V1  V4
II  aVL  V2  V5
III  aVF  V3  V6
II

25mm/s  10mm/mV  150Hz  003A-003A  12SL 250  CID: 2  EID:3  EDT: 13:35 02-JUN-1995  ORDER:

1–7  ECG during sinus rhythm from patient in example B (see text).

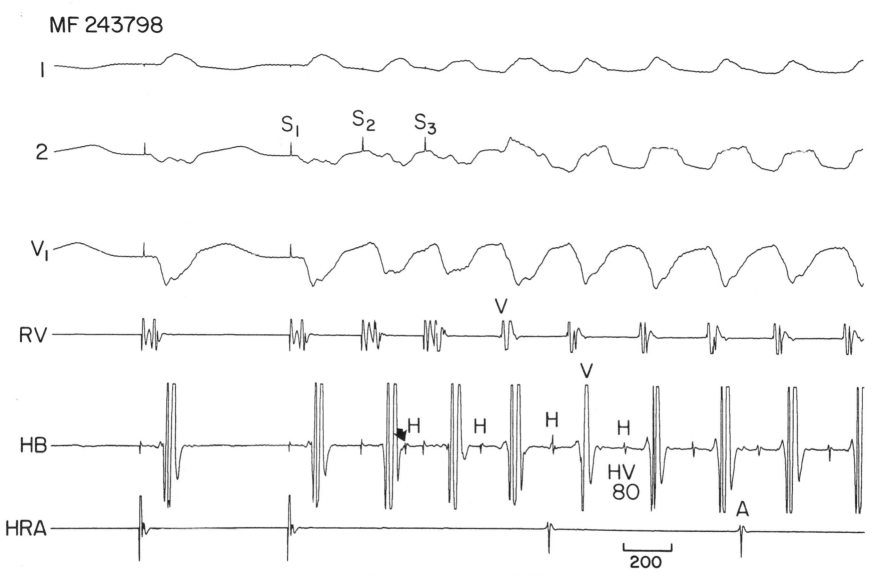

**1–8** Induction of tachycardia in patient from example B. The arrow indicates retrograde activation of the His bundle. HV, His-ventricular interval; $S_1$, last paced cycle of drive; $S_2$, $S_3$, extrastimuli.

MF 243798

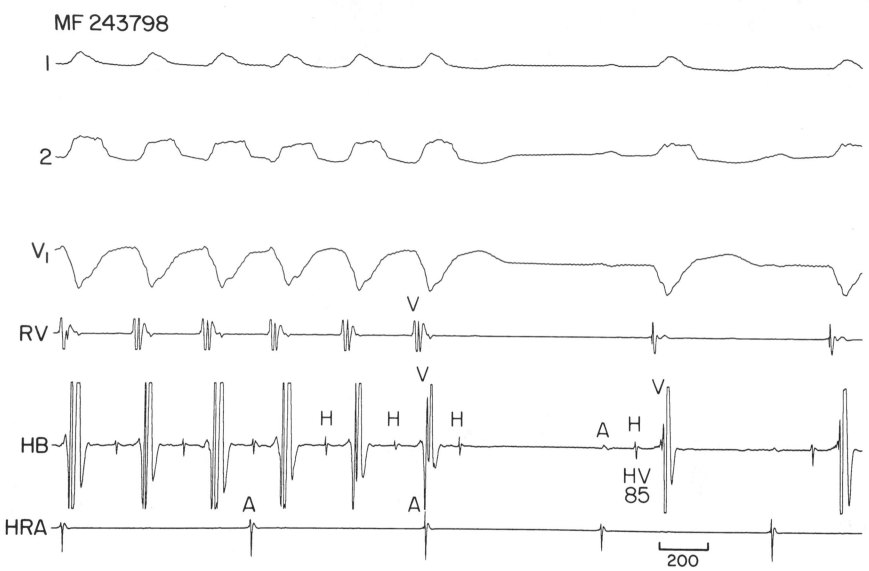

**1-9** Spontaneous termination of tachycardia in patient from example B.

**Table 1–4  Differential Diagnosis of Wide QRS Tachycardia**

- SVT tachycardia with aberrancy
- VT
- Preexcited tachycardia

**Table 1–5  Differential Diagnosis of Narrow QRS Tachycardia**

- Atrial tachycardia
- AV node reentry
- AV reentry
- Junctional tachycardia
- VT (fascicular tachycardia, "septal" VT can mimic SVT)

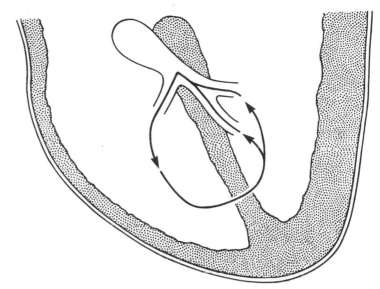

**A**

different rates, QRS morphology, and A–V relationship. The alternate hypothesis of one tachycardia mechanism with different manifestations is untenable.

The initial part of the trace has more atrial (A) electrograms than ventricular (V) electrograms with a variable atrial–ventricular (A–V) relationship and an atrial cycle length (CL) of 250 ms. This is atrial flutter.

The transition zone is marked by the arrow, the last flutter cycle. This is followed by a normal QRS that heralds the onset of the second tachycardia. The latter has left bundle branch block (LBBB) morphology and an apparent 1:1 A–V relationship. It is not clear whether the atria are driving the ventricles, whether the ventricles are driving the atria, or whether their relationship is reciprocal.

Atrial activation on the available leads begins at the proximal coronary sinus (CS) recording electrodes positioned near the orifice of the CS. This sequence is not discriminating, being compatible with atrial tachycardia, retrograde conduction over a "slow" AV node pathway, and retrograde conduction over an AP (see Table 1–6). The normal His ventricle (HV) relationship argues against ventricular tachycardia (VT) or preexcited tachycardia (see Table 1–8).

The differential diagnosis at this point includes atrial tachycardia,

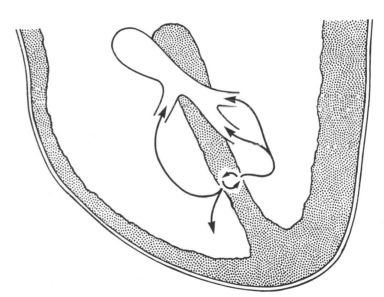

**B**

**1–10** Panel A shows schematic representation of bundle branch reentry. Panel B indicates intramyocardial reentry with passive activation of bundle branches. See text.

MF 243798

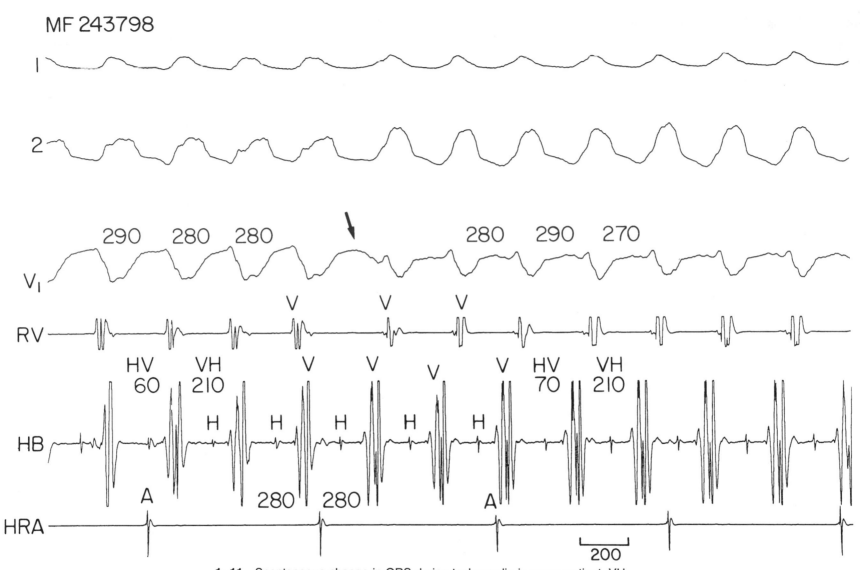

**1–11** Spontaneous change in QRS during tachycardia in same patient. VH, ventricular-His interval; cycle lengths in milliseconds.

**Table 1–6  Concentric Atrial Activation Sequence During Tachycardia**

- Narrow QRS complex
    - Atrial tachycardia
    - AV node reentry
    - AV reentry
    - Junctional tachycardia
- Wide QRS complex
    - SVT with aberrancy
    - Preexcited tachycardia
    - VT

**Table 1–7  Eccentric Atrial Activation Sequence During Tachycardia**

- Narrow QRS complex
    - Atrial tachycardia
    - AV reentry
- Wide QRS complex
    - SVT with aberrancy
    - Preexcited tachycardia
    - VT

**Table 1–8  Absent H or "Short" His Ventricle (HV) Interval During Tachycardia**

- VT
- Preexcited tachycardia
- Inappropriate His recording site

**Table 1–9  Preexcited Tachycardia: Concentric Atrial Activation**

- AP part of tachycardia circuit
    - Antidromic reentry (including atriofascicular type)
    - AP-to-AP reentry
    - Nodoventricular or nodofascicular reentry
- AP *not* part of tachycardia circuit ("bystander" conduction)
    - Atrial tachycardia
    - AV node reentry

**Table 1–10  Preexcited Tachycardia: Eccentric Atrial Activation**

- AP part of tachycardia circuit
    - AP-to-AP reentry
- AP *not* part of tachycardia circuit ("bystander" conduction)
    - Atrial tachycardia

**Table 1–11  Approach to Unknown EP Tracing**

- General overview
- Analyze the surface ECG
- Analyze the intracardiac records
- What is the *A to V relationship?*
- What is the *atrial activation sequence?*
- What is the *ventricular activation sequence* as determined from available sites?
- Is the His deflection visible and what is its relation to A and V? What are the apparent HV and VA intervals?
- Formulate a *hypothesis* and see if it explains all the observations.

atrioventricular reentry and atrioventricular node reentry. Atrioventricular reentry is favored over atrioventricular node reentry because there is only modest atrio-His (AH) prolongation at the onset and the VA interval is too long for the most common type of AV node reentry. More compellingly, the apparent VA interval prolongs by 60 ms with the development of LBBB aberration after the first tachycardia cycle, a situation only compatible with AV reentry utilizing a left lateral AP as part of the circuit. The remaining hypothesis of atrial tachycardia is not supported by the mode of onset or the apparent VA intervals, but is not yet ruled out entirely. It is important

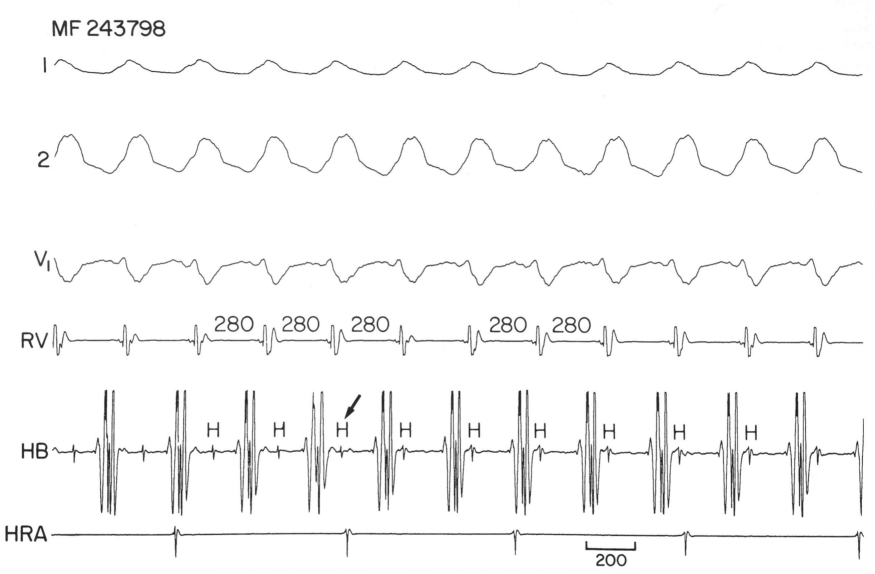

**1–12** Spontaneous change in timing of His deflection without change in QRS or cycle length in patient from example B.

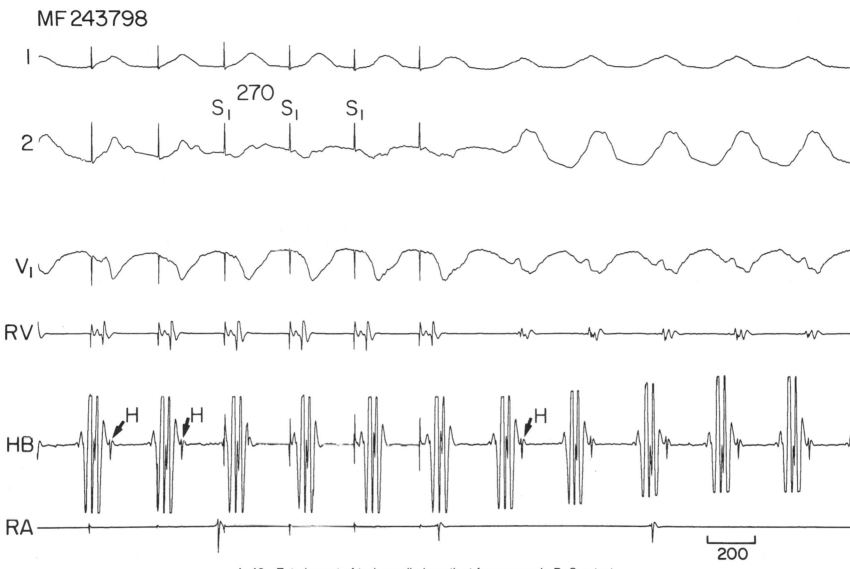

**1–13** Entrainment of tachycardia in patient from example B. See text.

to remember that the first atrial complex of the second tachycardia could have fortuitously started shortly after the last narrow QRS complex. Introduction of a relatively late-coupled premature ventricular complex (PVC) into the cardiac cycle at the time of His bundle refractoriness (Fig. 1–5) advances the next atrial cycle and terminates the tachycardia, verifying the diagnosis of AV reentry. We do appreciate that the patient could have had a concealed AP near an atrial tachycardia focus, with the PVC preexciting the atrium over the AP and terminating the atrial tachycardia. However, one does not need to look for zebras in a herd of horses!

### Example B

The patient is a 74-year-old man with a history of inferior and anterior myocardial infarction (MI) and coronary artery bypass grafting. He experiences the sudden onset of rapid heartbeating while watching television, and the ECG recorded subsequently in the emergency room is shown in Fig. 1–6. The arrhythmia stops spontaneously and the ECG recorded in sinus rhythm shows left bundle branch block (Fig. 1–7). Any wide QRS tachycardia in such a patient is presumptively VT, and this is supported by the suggestion of AV dissociation in the rhythm strip (*arrow*). However, the QRS during tachycardia is very similar, but not identical, to the QRS in sinus rhythm. VT with a QRS similar to the QRS during sinus rhythm may be seen with bundle branch reentry or VT originating in the His bundle (yes, the His bundle is a ventricular structure). Alternatively, VT originating in the fasicular system or adjacent myocardium could be expected to break out at the same site as the sinus impulse in the presence of bundle branch block. Thus, the EP study is begun with a differential diagnosis of bundle branch reentry or fascicular VT high on the list.

At EP study, tachycardia is induced with two ventricular extrastimuli (Fig. 1–8) and terminates spontaneously (Fig. 1–9). Atrioventricular dissociation is now clearly evident and the QRS in sinus rhythm is again similar to tachycardia. The tachycardia begins with prolongation of the retrograde His bundle (H) and the HV during tachycardia is similar to that in sinus rhythm. This is most compatible with bundle branch reentry as illustrated in Fig. 1–10 (panel A),

although the alternative hypothesis (Fig. 1–10, panel B) is not disproved. The diagnosis is further supported by the ventricular activation sequence that shows very early activation of the right ventricular apex (near the terminus of the right bundle branch). Spontaneous termination with a retrograde H is compatible with either hypothesis.

Is there enough evidence to proceed with ablation of the right bundle branch? A further induction of tachycardia is pursued (Fig. 1–11) and a spontaneous transition to another QRS morphology (*arrow*) is observed. In spite of a clear change in the QRS (although still LBBB morphology) and ventricular activation sequence (the RV apex is now very late), the tachycardia rate and the H electrogram are unchanged! Consider the two hypotheses in Fig. 1–10. The evident loss of anterograde right bundle activation (as assumed by the relatively late activation of the right ventricular apical electrogram) was not critical to maintenance of tachycardia and the right bundle was clearly a bystander. Further observation of the tachycardia (Fig. 1–12) illustrates another transition (*arrow*). The ventricular-His (VH) interval shortens to a new steady state and again the tachycardia rate remains unchanged, oblivious to activity in the H. It is now obvious that the H and right bundle are passive bystanders and the tachycardia is best explained by myocardial reentry with passive activation of the bundle branches (Fig. 1–10B).

What if we were not fortunate enough to see the phenomena in Figs. 1–11 and 1–12? Entraining VT by pacing the right ventricular apex (Fig. 1–13) at a cycle length only 20 ms shorter than the VT cycle length advances the retrograde H by 50 ms or more, dynamically dissociating the H from the tachycardia circuit.

The unknown tracings in the following chapters provide an opportunity to practice these principles. A question after each trace is intended to focus attention on the intended point of interest although the tracings usually provide other lessons. Measuring calipers and a clear right angle for vertical alignment are recommended. Finally, there may well be alternative explanations for phenomena to the ones suggested. Dr. Charles Fisch once responded to a contrary student at an ECG course by saying that his explanation was correct because it was his slide. We can say it no better.

# Chapter 2
# Fundamentals of
# Clinical Electrophysiology

## *Figure 2–1A*

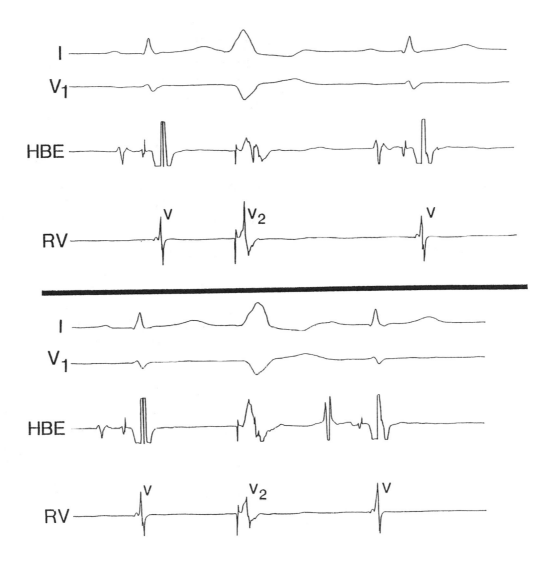

A series of interpolated PVCs was introduced in this patient during sinus rhythm. What is the effect of the PVC on conduction of the subsequent sinus complex? What is this called? Why is conduction of the sinus complex of the PVC different in the upper and lower panels?

# Figure 2-1B

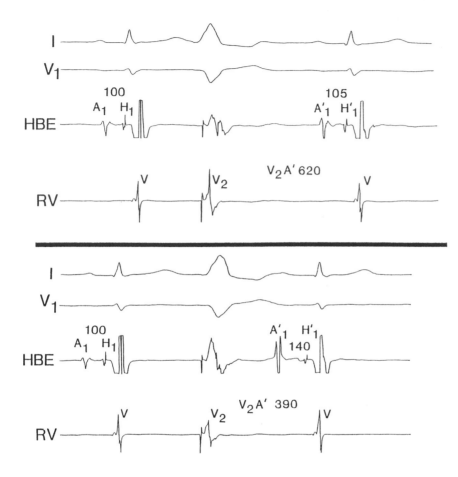

## Explanation:

The electrophysiologic phenomenon exhibited is *concealed conduction*. Concealed conduction occurs because the PVC conducts retrogradely into the AV node but not to the atrium, and conduction into the AV node is not visible (concealed). The result is prolongation of AV nodal refractoriness. The sinus complex after the PVC has an increase of the AH interval from 100 to 105 ms (upper panel). This increase in AH interval would likely be missed during analysis of the surface electrocardiogram performed at 25 mm/s paper speed. It is, however, demonstrated during intracardiac measurements performed at faster paper speeds. Conduction of the PVC into the AV node is confirmed because of the subsequent prolongation of AV node conduction.

The effects of concealed conduction are more prominent in the lower panel. Note that the AH interval after the PVC is 140 ms compared with 105 ms in the upper panel. The longer AH interval occurs because the PVC is introduced later in diastole and consequently closer to the next sinus complex. There is less recovery of AV nodal excitability as a consequence. Note that the $V_2A'$ in the upper panel is 620 ms but only 390 ms in the lower panel. This demonstrates the well-known inverse relationship of the effect of PVCs on PR and RP intervals as identified in the electrocardiogram. In other words, as a PVC occurs closer to the next sinus P wave (short RP), there is a more marked effect on subsequent PR prolongation or even block. This relationship is identified in Fig. 2–1C. As $V_2A_1'$ shortens, $A_1'H_1'$ progressively lengthens until block of the subsequent sinus complex occurs.

## *Figure 2–1C*

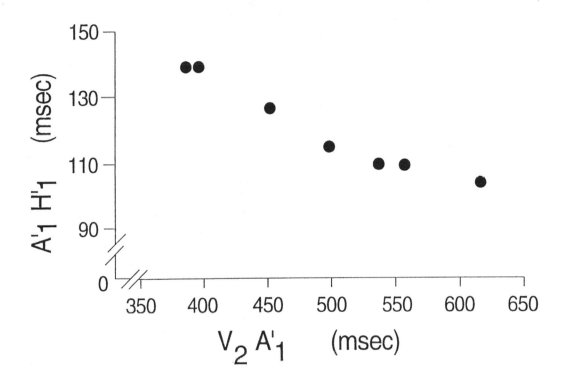

# Figure 2-2A

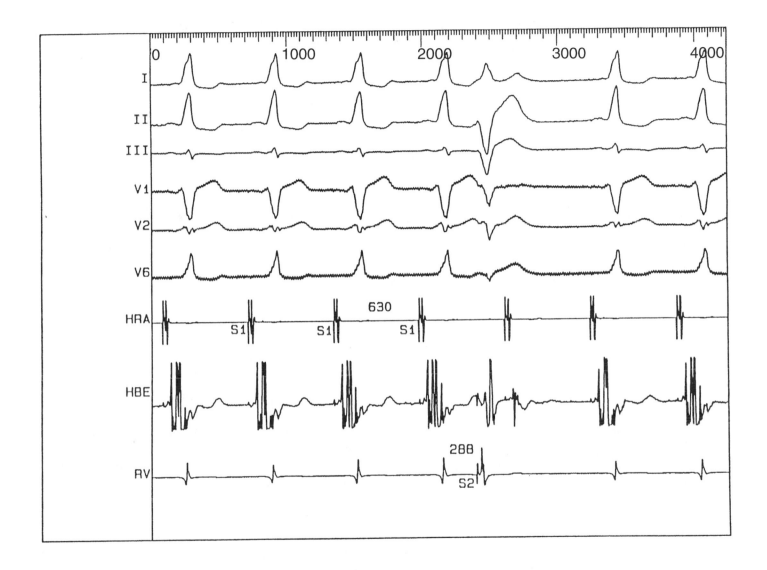

This patient with a history of tachycardia had a PVC introduced during atrial pacing at CL 630-ms. What EP phenomenon occurs after the PVC? What is the most likely cause of this patient's tachycardia?

## Figure 2–2B

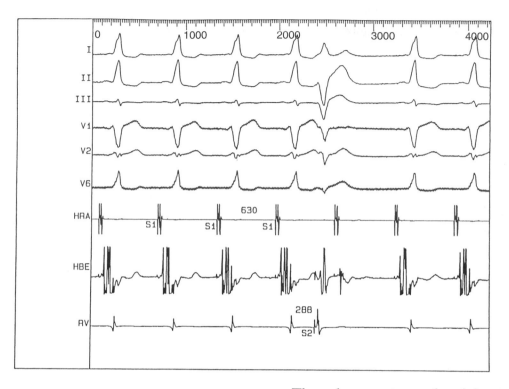

**Explanation:**

During atrial pacing the ECG leads demonstrate a relatively short PR interval with a wide QRS complex. Analysis of the His bundle electrogram reveals continuous electrical activity with the atrial and ventricular electrograms appearing to merge into one another. No clearly defined His deflection is seen. These two observations strongly imply the wide QRS complex is due to ventricular preexcitation with conduction over an AP. The fact that there is almost continuous electrical activity identified on the His bundle electrogram suggests, but does not prove, the AP is in the vicinity of the His bundle recording site. Statistically, the most likely tachycardia would be AV reentry, although patients with ventricular preexcitation are not immune to other forms of tachyarrhythmias.

The subsequent paced atrial complex after the PVC ($S_2$) does not conduct to the ventricle. Thus, retrograde concealed conduction has occurred not only into the normal ventriculoatrial conduction system but also into the AP. Otherwise, one would have expected the atrial paced complex to conduct over the AP, which does not occur. A much less likely but alternative explanation for lack of AP conduction is refractoriness of the ventricle after the PVC. We think this is extremely unlikely since the anticipated ventricular activation over the AP would have occurred more than 300 ms after the PVC was introduced. There should be more than sufficient time for ventricular repolarization to have occurred, and the ventricle should be excitable if the AP is capable of conduction.

## Figure 2–3A

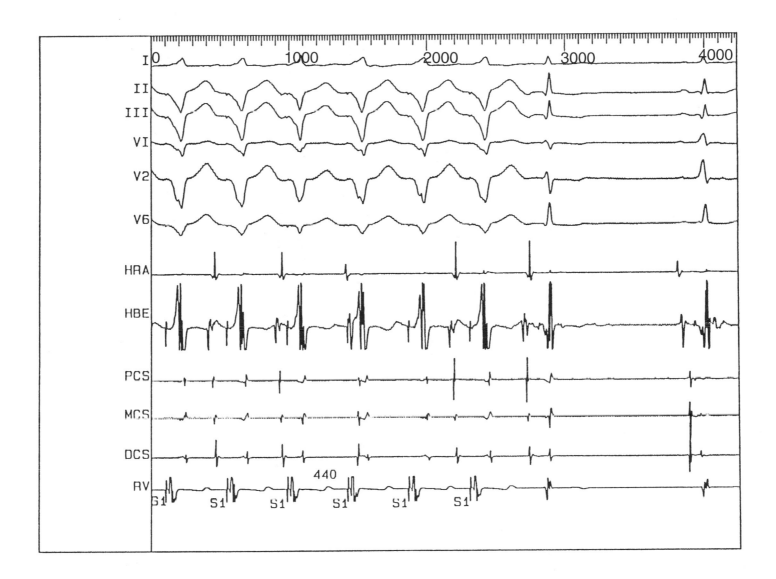

Retrograde Wenckebach block occurs during ventricular pacing at
440-ms CL. What is the likely mechanism for block?

## Figure 2-3B

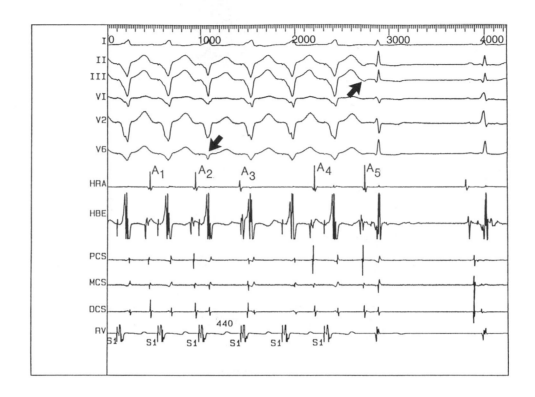

**Explanation:**

Apparent Wenckebach ventriculoatrial (VA) block occurs because of reentry in the AV node. Analysis of the surface electrocardiogram reveals a shortened QRS duration following $A_2$ (*arrow*). This ventricular fusion occurs because a portion of the ventricle is activated by an electrical wavefront differing from that produced during pacing alone. The third paced ventricular complex is also associated with VA block. $A_3$ has a different intracardiac activation sequence from $A_1$ and $A_2$, and the high right atrial electrogram precedes the septal atrial electrogram noted in the His bundle lead. This may be a premature atrial complex or less likely sinus capture. Analysis of $A_4$ and $A_5$ reveals the AV nodal echo complex. Note the marked increase in VA conduction time for $A_5$ with a retrograde P wave (*arrow*) in ECG lead III. Pacing was terminated and the echo became manifest as the ventricle was activated with a narrow QRS complex. Anterograde conduction of this echo complex precludes retrograde conduction over the AV node and therefore block occurs. The fusion complex noted by the arrow in ECG lead $V_6$ can be explained by ventricular activation over the normal AV node/His-Purkinje system (HPS) and the ventricular paced complex. Note that $A_2$-QRS and $A_5$-QRS conduction times are very similar.

# Figure 2–4A

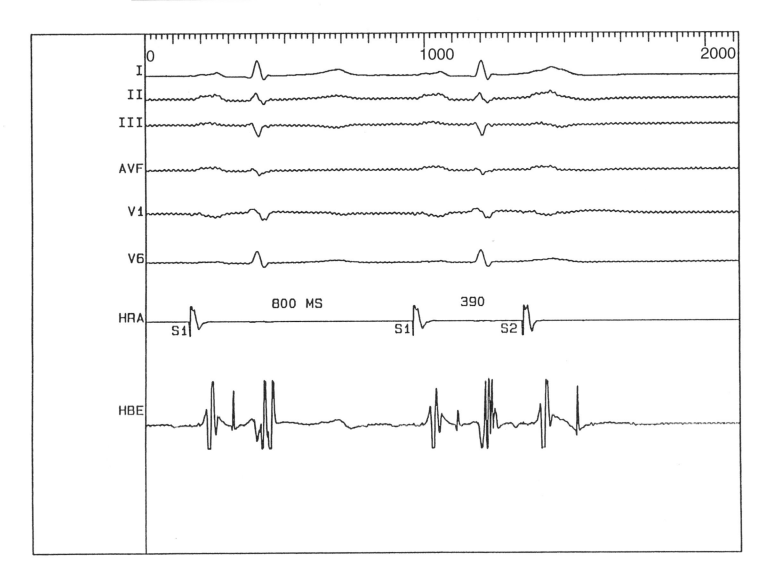

Figures 2–4A and B were recorded during an EP study of a patient with syncope. What EP phenomenon is present? Does this patient need a pacemaker?

# Figure 2–4B

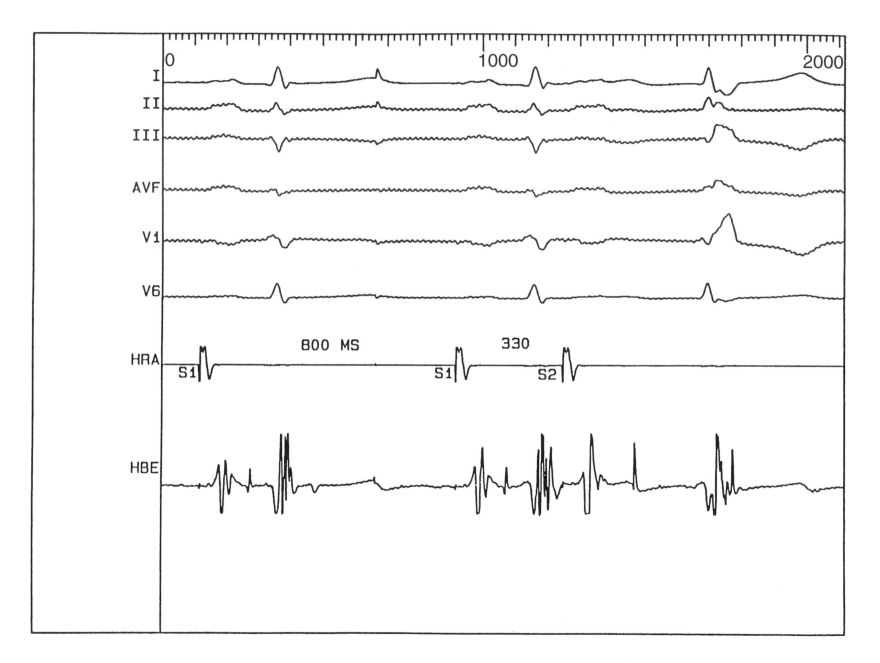

# Figure 2–4C

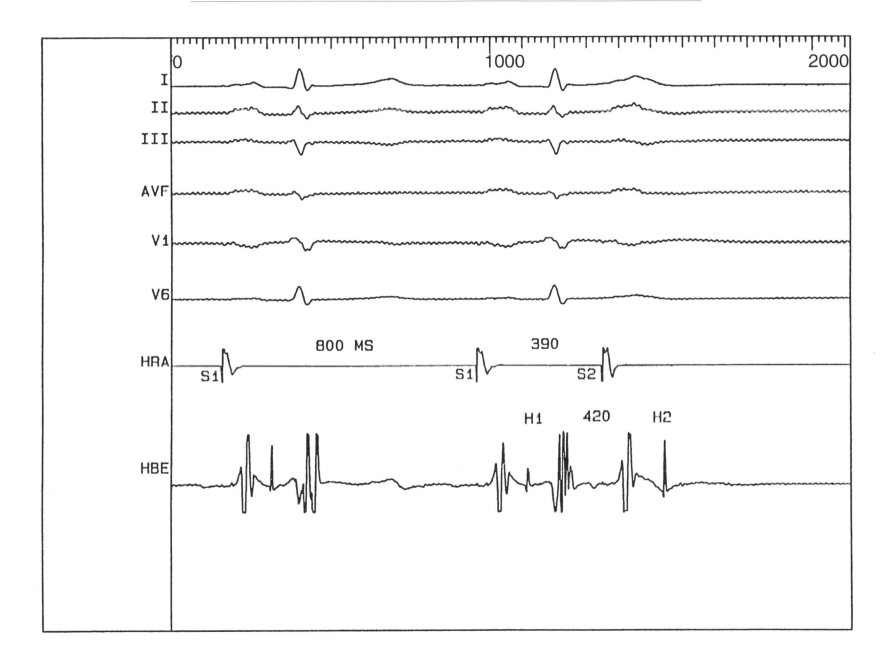

# Figure 2–4D

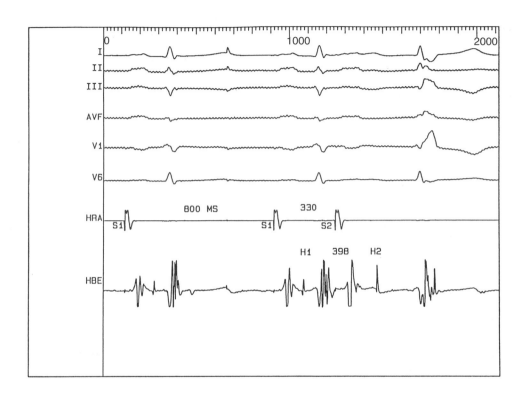

## Explanation:

The electrophysiologic phenomenon is conduction GAP. Figure 2–4C demonstrates block below the His bundle recording site of a premature atrial complex of 390 ms. A narrow QRS complex occurs during atrial paced CL 800 ms. The $H_1H_2$ interval is 420 ms, which is probably within normal limits at this heart rate. This patient has excellent AV nodal conduction and therefore a relatively short $H_1H_2$ interval could be achieved. This is not an abnormal finding and is certainly not an indication for a pacemaker.

In Fig. 2–4D, a shorter premature atrial complex of 330 ms conducts to the ventricle with right bundle branch block (RBBB) morphology. The $H_1H_2$ interval is shorter in Fig. 2–4D compared with Fig. 2–4C. Note the marked prolongation of His-Purkinje conduction time ($H_2V$) in this complex compared with the normal His-Purkinje conduction time of $S_1$. Conduction at the shorter premature atrial interval and block at the longer premature atrial interval is an example of gap physiology. Gap occurs because the more premature atrial complex exhibits slower conduction proximal to the previous site of block; this allows subsequent recovery of excitability of that area and conduction to the ventricle. In this instance gap occurred in the HPS as noted by block initially after the recorded $H_2$ potential. Subsequent conduction has marked slowing of infra-His conduction time.

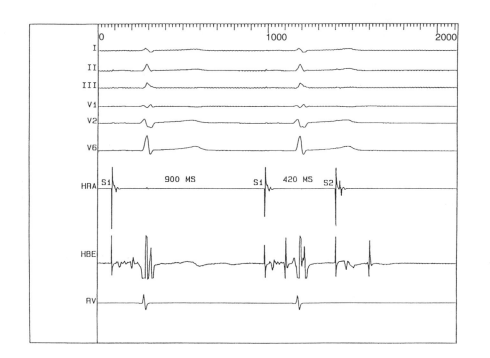

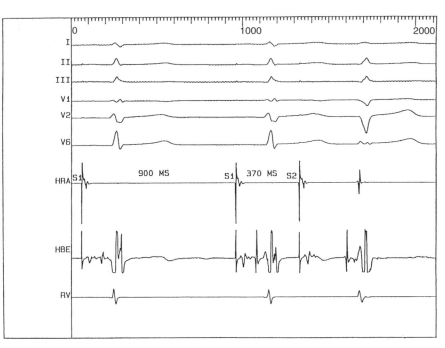

This patient was being studied because of SVT. What EP phenomenon occurs and what is the likely cause of tachycardia?

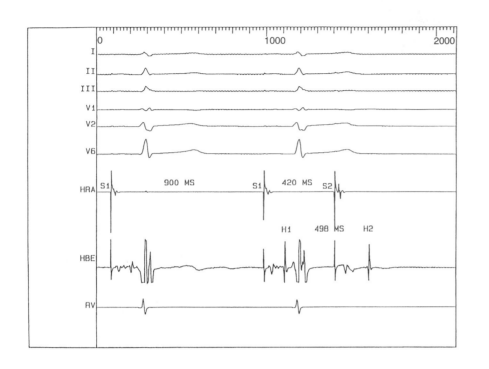

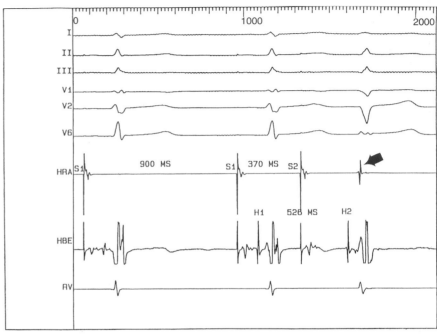

## Explanation:

During atrial pacing at a slow rate of 900 ms, a premature atrial complex of 420 ms blocked below the His bundle recording (Fig. 2–5C). Note that $H_1H_2$ is 498 ms, which is relatively long. Regardless, block below the His bundle recording in this situation should not be considered abnormal and does not require pacemaker implantation. In Fig. 2–5D, there is resumption of conduction with a shorter premature atrial coupling interval of 370 ms. However, there is a substantial prolongation of $H_1H_2$ interval to 526 ms and the con-

ducted QRS complex has a relatively normal HV interval with incomplete LBBB. Thus, there is some delay in conduction in the left bundle branch system. This example of gap occurs in the AV node, with resumption of conduction resulting primarily from an increase in AH interval of the $S_2$. Note also the retrograde atrial complex (*arrow*). This is an AV nodal echo and strongly suggests that the patient has AV node reentry as the cause of tachycardia. This echo complex did not conduct subsequently to the AV node, but AV node reentry was easily initiated during isoproterenol infusion that allowed facilitation of anterograde AV node conduction.

## *Figure 2–6A*

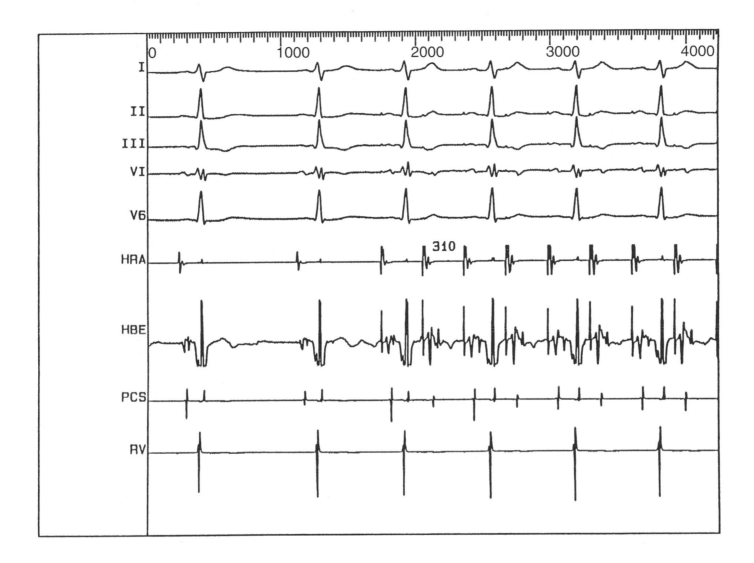

This patient underwent EP study because of syncope. Atrial pacing was initiated at a relatively short CL of 310 ms. Where does block occur? Is this abnormal? Does the patient require pacemaker therapy?

## Figure 2-6B

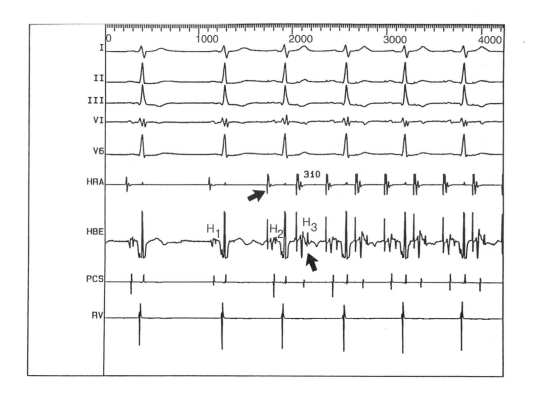

### Explanation:

This patient has a relatively slow sinus CL of approximately 900 ms. Atrial pacing is initiated suddenly at a cycle length of 310 ms. The first paced atrial complex (arrow on the HRA lead) conducts to the ventricle. The $H_1H_2$ interval noted on the His bundle lead is still relatively long and conduction occurs without any problem. The second atrial complex blocks below a recorded His potential (*arrow;* $H_3$). The $H_2H_3$ interval is short and follows a relatively long $H_1H_2$ interval. Then, 2:1 block occurs below the recorded His potential for the rest of this tracing. This is a normal finding that happens because of the preceding slow CL before rapid atrial pacing. The long CL results in prolongation of His-Purkinje refractoriness, and the short $H_2H_3$ interval occurs within the absolute refractory period of the His-Purkinje system. Thus, block occurs below the recorded $H_3$ deflection, a normal finding. A pacemaker is not required. In this same patient, a gradual increase in atrial pacing rate to CL 310 ms produced 1:1 AV conduction. This was due to the progressive shortening of His-Purkinje refractoriness as the rate was incrementally increased, rather than an abrupt increase in heart rate.

# Figure 2–7A

## During Sleep

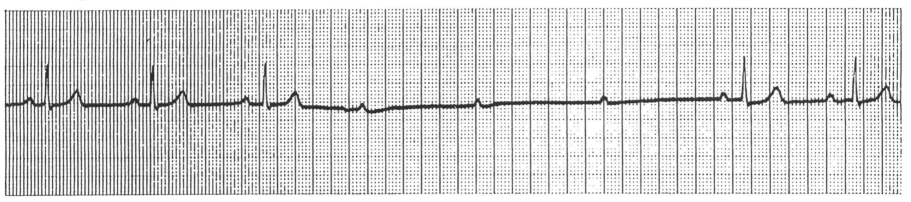

This tracing occurred during in-hospital telemetry monitoring. There is no history of syncope or presyncope. Does this patient require electrophysiologic testing? Should a pacemaker be implanted?

## *Figure 2–7B*

# During Sleep

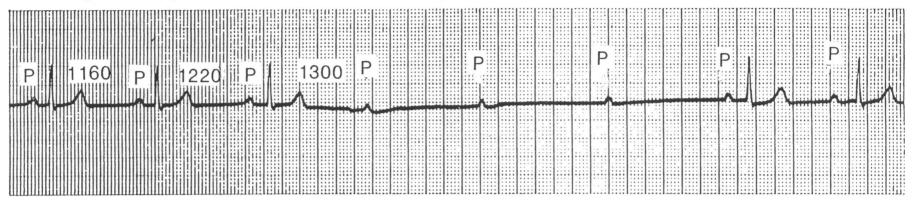

**Explanation:**

This recording was made while the patient was sleeping. Note that there is progressive increase in the PP interval until block occurs. In addition, there is the unusual finding of several blocked P waves prior to a junctional escape or conducted complex, a distinction impossible to determine from the data presented. The progressive prolongation of PP intervals prior to a nonconducted P wave strongly suggests a vagal mechanism as the cause of AV block. The heightened vagal tone could explain both slowing of sinus node automaticity and AV node block. Although it cannot be proven by this tracing, block invariably occurs in the AV node in this situation. This is a relatively common occurrence during Holter recordings or in-hospital telemetry monitoring. Distinctly unusual is the high-grade AV block noted in this patient. However, in the absence of any symptoms of syncope or presyncope, this patient does not require EP testing or an implanted pacemaker. A workup for sleep apnea may be useful.

## *Figure 2–8A*

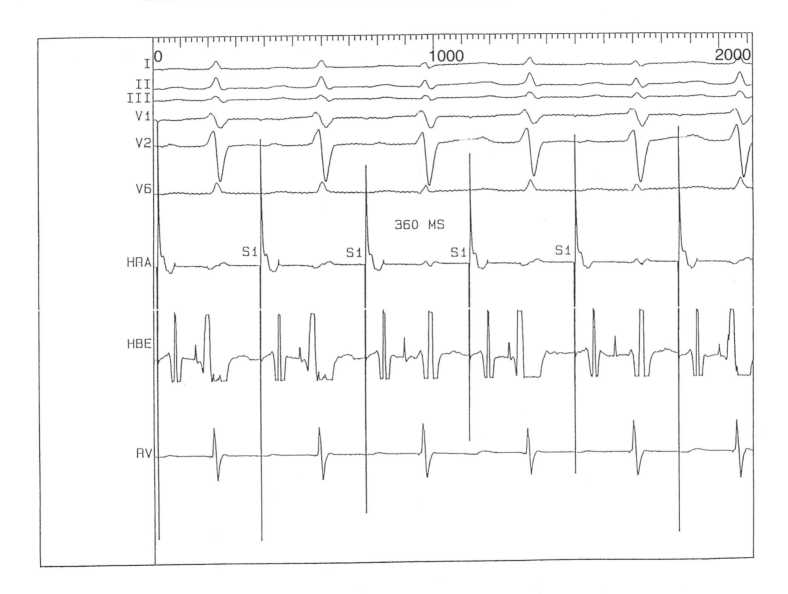

This tracing was taken during an EP study during atrial pacing at
CL 360 ms. What is the diagnosis?

# Figure 2–8B

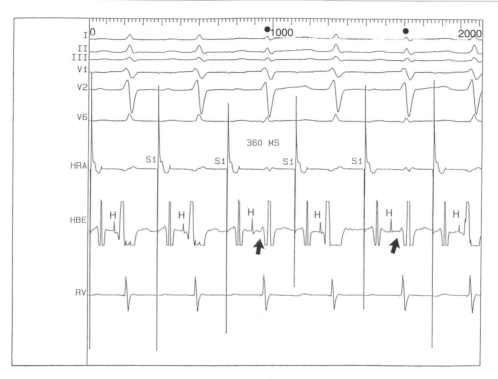

## Explanation:

This patient had SVT due to AV reentry using an AP for retrograde conduction. After successful ablation of the AP a repeat EP study was performed. During incremental atrial pacing there was a sudden change in the AV interval as noted in Fig. 2–8B. Note that the arrow reveals a sudden lengthening of the HV interval that occurred in a 2:1 conduction pattern for several complexes. In addition, the QRS complexes with a filled dot on top reveal a different morphology from the rest of the QRS complexes. This is a very unusual finding, and the shorter HV intervals without the arrow occur because of conduction over a fasciculoventricular AP. This diagnosis is made by the subtle preexcitation noted in the QRS complexes associated with a shorter than expected HV interval. The degree of preexcitation is minimal since the ventricle is activated over an AP that connects the bundle branch system with the ventricle. Thus, there is minimal time to preexcite the ventricle compared with conduction over the normal AV conduction system.

It would be extremely difficult to diagnose a fasciculoventricular AP unless block occurred revealing the normal HV interval, as happened here. One could argue that the shorter HV intervals are actually not His deflections but right bundle branch deflections, and the true HV interval is noted by the complexes with an arrow. However, a right bundle branch potential typically occurs with a smaller atrial electrogram compared with the atrial electrogram recorded with the His bundle. In the former situation the catheter is situated more distally nearer to the ventricle. In this tracing, there is no significant change in atrial amplitude for any of the paced complexes. In addition, this would not explain the subtle but real change in the QRS complex that occurs with the longer HV interval. These observations are best explained by the presence of a fasciculoventricular AP.

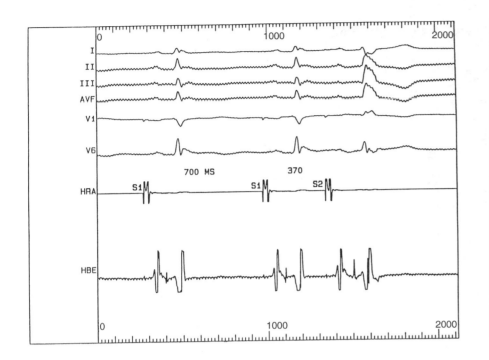

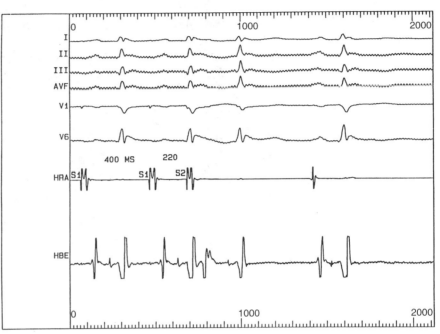

During the EP study in this patient, premature atrial complexes (PACs) were introduced at paced CL 700 ms (Fig. 2–9A) and 400 ms (Fig. 2–9B). What occurs and why?

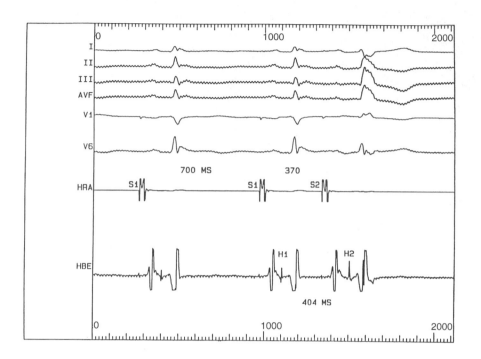

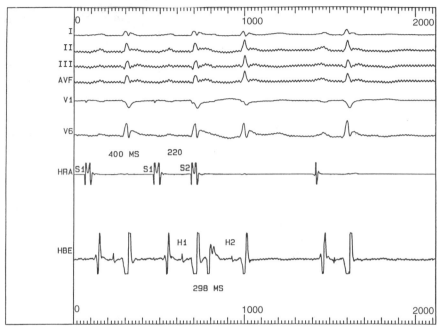

## Explanation:

Figure 2–9*C* demonstrates high right atrial pacing at 700 ms with a PAC introduced at 370 ms. This results in an $H_1H_2$ interval of 404 ms and a RBBB pattern. All longer $H_1H_2$ intervals were conducted with a normal QRS complex. Thus, the refractory period of the right bundle branch is 404 ms. By electrocardiographic criteria, this is a RBBB pattern. However, actual block in the right bundle branch does not have to occur in this situation. Instead, there could be slowed conduction in the right bundle branch relative to the left bundle branch, allowing delayed activation of the right ventricle with a RBBB pattern. Thus, a RBBB block morphology can represent either marked slowing of conduction or actual block in the right bundle branch.

Figure 2–9*D* occurs during high right atrial pacing at CL 400 ms with a markedly shorter premature atrial interval than noted in Fig. 2–9*C*. The resulting $H_1H_2$ interval is considerably shorter but right bundle branch conduction occurs. This demonstrates the effect of heart rate on bundle branch refractoriness. At slower heart rates the refractoriness of the HPS is relatively longer compared with faster heart rates. In this example, RBBB refractoriness is less than 298 ms at a heart rate of 150 beats/min (Fig. 2–9*D*) but is 404 ms at a heart rate of 86 beats/min (Fig. 2–9*C*). These effects of heart rate on bundle branch refractoriness are commonly manifested during continuous electrocardiographic recordings. Typically, a PAC with aberrancy occurs during slow rates but, when the heart rate is faster, a PAC with a similar coupling interval conducts with a narrow QRS.

# *Figure 2–10A*

## Control

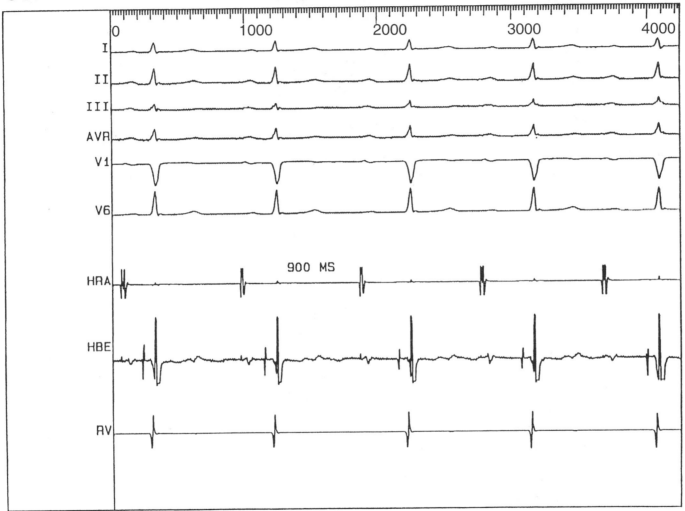

This recording was obtained during study of a patient with a history of SVT. What is the most likely cause of tachycardia in this individual?

# Figure 2-10B

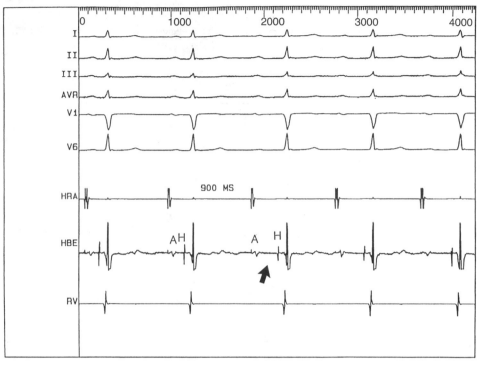

## Explanation:

During fixed atrial pacing at CL 900 ms there is a sudden prolongation in the PR interval that stays relatively fixed. The arrow demonstrates the marked sudden prolongation in AH interval compared with the previous shorter AH interval. When a sudden and unexpected prolongation in PR interval, or AH interval, occurs and remains relatively fixed, the likely diagnosis is dual AV nodal physiology. In this example, the first two atrial paced complexes conduct to the ventricle with a much shorter PR and AH interval than the subsequent complexes because conduction proceeds over the fast pathway of the AV node. The third atrial complex has a sudden prolongation of the PR and AH interval because block occurred over the fast AV nodal pathway and conduction now proceeds over the slow AV nodal pathway. The demonstration of dual AV nodal physiology in a patient with documented paroxysmal SVT strongly suggests AV node reentry is the cause of tachycardia. In fact, with intravenous isoproterenol, AV node reentry was initiated.

The demonstration of dual AV nodal physiology can be recognized occasionally during routine electrocardiography or continuous electrocardiographic recordings. If there is a sudden, unexpected, constant prolongation of the PR interval that does not progress to block, one should strongly suspect dual AV node physiology. This does not suggest that the patient has or will develop tachycardia since the patient may lack retrograde AV nodal conduction, which typically precludes AV node reentry. Thus, to initiate the slow/fast variety of AV node reentry there must be *both* anterograde block in the fast pathway and subsequent retrograde conduction over this pathway.

# Figure 2–11A and 2–11B

**Resting ECG**

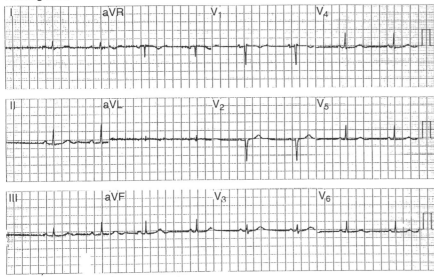

A middle-age woman presented with exercise-induced presyncope. Her resting ECG (left) and ECG lead II rhythm strips during exercise (right) are shown. Is conduction delay and block most likely to occur in the AV node, His bundle, or bundle branch system?

## A. Standing

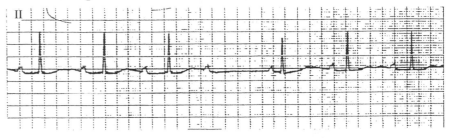

## B. Stage 3 TM

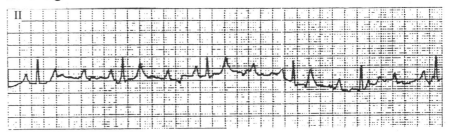

## C. Recovery

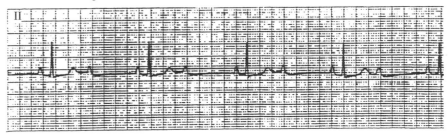

# Figure 2-11C

**Figure 2-11C**

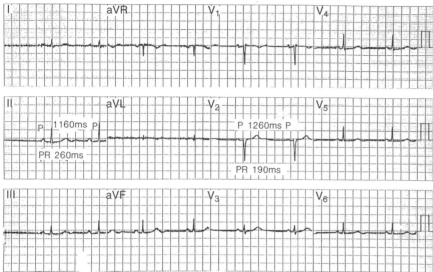

**Resting ECG**

*Explanation:*

Figure 2-11C demonstrates the resting ECG with variable PR intervals. Note that during the beginning of the tracing in lead II with a sinus cycle length (SCL) of 1160 ms the PR interval is 260 ms. Later in the tracing as shown in V₂ the SCL is 1260 ms with a PR interval of 190 ms. Ideally, one should measure changes using the same ECG lead, but the PR differences are obvious. The QRS complex is narrow, suggesting lack of significant disease in the bundle branch system. However, this certainly does not exclude disease within the His bundle that may occur without bundle branch block. From this electrocardiogram alone, it is difficult to determine the site of variable conduction. However, one should suspect disease in the His bundle. Shortening of the SCL is likely due to autonomic changes such as decreased vagal tone or increased sympathetic tone, both of which usually improve conduction through the AV node.

Figure 2-11D shows the tracings from the treadmill evaluation and highlights the effect of heart rate on AV conduction. When the patient was standing (panel A), the SCL shortened to 1020 ms and this resulted in type 1 second-degree AV block. As the SCL progressively decreased during the treadmill test, the degree of conduction block increased; for example, 3:1 conduction in stage 3 of the treadmill with a SCL of 440 ms (panel B). During recovery (panel C), the SCL progressively lengthened to 860 ms and 2:1 conduction occurred. At this time the phenomenon of ventriculophasic sinus arrhythmia is noted (see below). The autonomic effects of standing and exercise are parasympathetic withdrawal and increased sympathetic tone. These combined changes decrease SCL. They also facilitate AV node conduction. Thus, the paradoxical effect of decreased SCL producing progressively worse AV conduction strongly implicates the HPS as the site of conduction problems. The narrow QRS complex implies lack of bundle branch disease and the assumption is that conduction abnormalities occur within the His bundle. There was no need to perform an EP evaluation in this patient since the cause of her symptoms was identified during treadmill testing. In

# Figure 2–11D

## A. Standing

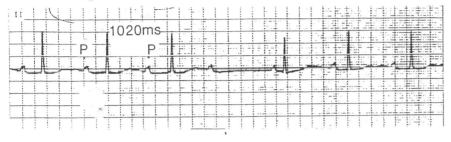

## B. Stage 3 TM

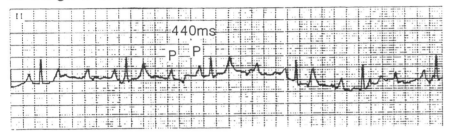

## C. Recovery

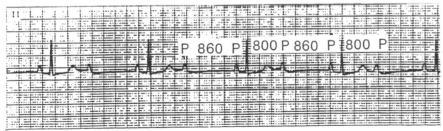

other patients we have correlated intra-His block in similar circumstances. This patient required a dual chamber pacemaker and symptoms abated after its implantation.

**Ventriculophasic Sinus Arrhythmia**

During recovery there is 2 : 1 conduction (Fig. 2–11D). There is also an interesting pattern of longer PP intervals between QRS complexcs compared with shorter PP intervals that surround a QRS complex. The mechanism for this ventriculophasic sinus arrhythmia is in part due to alternations in sinus nodal automaticity secondary to changes in blood pressure. Each QRS complex is associated with an increase in blood pressure, which affects the baroreceptors. Onc needs to postulate that the baroreceptor-mediated slowing of the sinus rate occurs too latc to affect the P wave immediately after the QRS complex, but does prolong the subsequent SCL. Thus, the PP interval between the two QRS complexes is lengthened. Because the effect of heightened blood pressure is short lived, the P wave immediately after the QRS complex is not delayed, resulting in a shortened PP interval surrounding the QRS complex.

*Figure 2–12A*

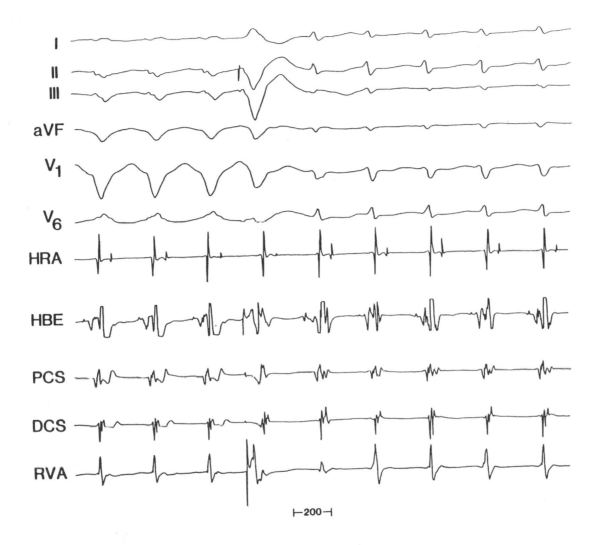

I

II

III

aVF

V₁

V₆

HRA

HBE

PCS

DCS

RVA

⊢200⊣

This patient has a history of wide and narrow QRS complex tachycardia. This tracing was taken during an EP study. What is the most likely diagnosis? What is the most likely mechanism for transformation from the wide QRS complex to the narrow QRS complex during tachycardia?

# Figure 2–12B

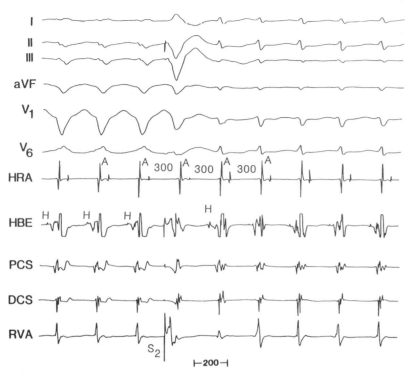

### Explanation:

The tachycardia mechanism is similar during bundle branch block aberrancy or normal QRS morphology. The short VA interval, identified as an atrial ECG within the QRS complex, rules out AV reentry. The long AH interval and relatively short HA and VA intervals are consistent with AV node reentry. From this tracing alone, an atrial tachycardia cannot be excluded, but this would be a far less likely diagnosis. In this situation one would have to postulate an atrial tachycardia with conduction over a slow pathway. This patient had AV node reentry.

The first three QRS complexes demonstrate typical LBBB morphology. Note in the His bundle lead that a small His deflection is present and the HV interval is similar to that recorded with the subsequent narrow QRS complexes. Thus, the first three QRS complexes represent LBBB aberrancy. There is minimal to no difference in the tachycardia cycle length between LBBB and narrow QRS complex morphology. It is therefore highly unlikely that LBBB aberrancy is due to an acceleration-dependent mechanism. The persistence of LBBB aberrancy is typical for transseptal concealed conduction. In this situation, a supraventricular complex conducts to the ventricle over the right bundle branch and blocks over the left bundle branch. Then, transseptal concealed conduction (not visible) occurs from the right to left ventricle with retrograde invasion of the impulse into the distal left bundle branch. This relatively late activation of the left bundle branch will prolong its refractoriness compared with the right bundle branch. When the next supraventricular impulse arrives at the left bundle branch it will be refractory and block occurs. This sequence persists and LBBB aberrancy continues with each tachycardia cycle. A similar scenario can occur with persistent RBBB aberrancy due to retrograde invasion from the left bundle branch into the right bundle branch distally.

Introduction of a PVC ($S_2$) during tachycardia at a critical coupling interval can result in termination of the transseptal concealed conduction. The premature ventricular complex "peels" back the refractory period of the left bundle branch by preventing the impulse from the right bundle branch from activating it at its usual later time. In other words, the PVC activates the left bundle branch earlier than would have been anticipated had the right bundle branch caused retrograde activation of this structure. Now, when the next supraventricular impulse reaches the left bundle branch anterogradely, it will conduct without block and this ends the persistence of bundle branch block aberrancy. In summary, this patient has typical AV node reentry with anterograde conduction over the slow pathway and retrograde conduction over the fast pathway. LBBB aberrancy occurred during the initiation of tachycardia and persisted until a PVC was introduced. LBBB aberrancy was caused by transseptal concealed conduction from the right bundle branch into the distal left bundle branch. This sequence was interrupted with the PVC that peeled back refractoriness of the left bundle branch and allowed the next supraventricular impulse to conduct normally over both bundle branches.

# Figure 2–13A

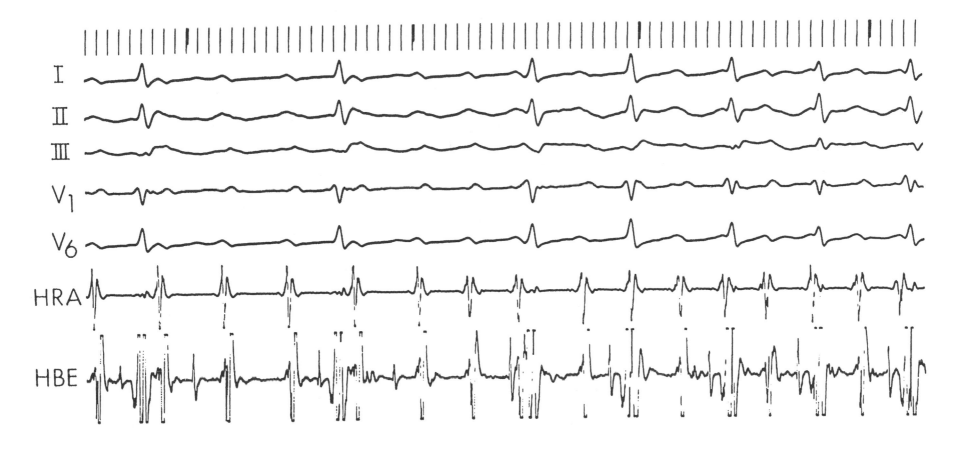

This tachycardia was initiated at EP study performed approximately
1 week after surgical ablation of an AP many years ago. Where does
AV block occur? Does this patient require permanent pacing? Time
lines on top are 50 ms.

## *Figure 2–13B*

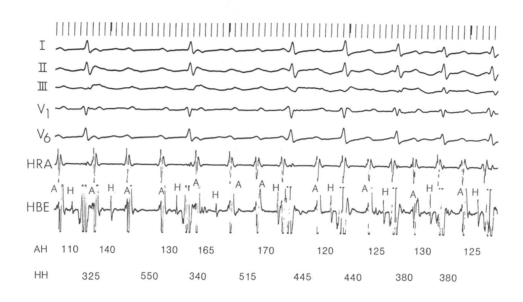

| AH | 110 | 140 | 130 | 165 | 170 | 120 | 125 | 130 | 125 |
|----|-----|-----|-----|-----|-----|-----|-----|-----|-----|

| HH | 325 | 550 | 340 | 515 | 445 | 440 | 380 | 380 |
|----|-----|-----|-----|-----|-----|-----|-----|-----|

### *Explanation:*

An atrial tachycardia was initiated at EP study, which was not a clinical arrhythmia for this patient. However, an interesting EP phenomenon occurred with AV block in both the AV node and HPS. On the left-hand portion of the figure AV nodal Wenckebach block occurs with an increase in the AH interval from 110 to 140 ms before block. Note the lack of a His bundle deflection after the third atrial electrogram. The fourth atrial electrogram demonstrates an AH interval of 130 ms and another Wenckebach AV nodal conduction pattern occurs. Then, the patient develops 2:1 AV conduction with a change in atrial rate.

The AV nodal Wenckebach conduction pattern produced variable HH intervals, which is physiologic. The changes in HH intervals result in block below the recorded His deflection. Block occurs with the shorter HH cycle immediately after a relatively long HH interval that results in prolongation of His-Purkinje refractoriness. Analysis of the sequence starting with the HH interval of 550 ms reveals that the subsequent HH interval is 340 ms and block occurs below the His deflection. The next HH interval is 515 ms, but now there is 2:1 block. This allows a relatively long HH interval of 445 ms and the subsequent HH intervals are similarly prolonged enough to allow conduction with each His deflection. The second atrial complex demonstrates block below the His bundle deflection and it is presumed that this HH interval of 325 ms was preceded by a relatively long HH interval, although this is not shown in the tracing. Infra-His block that results from a long–short HH sequence is physiologic. No pacemaker is required.

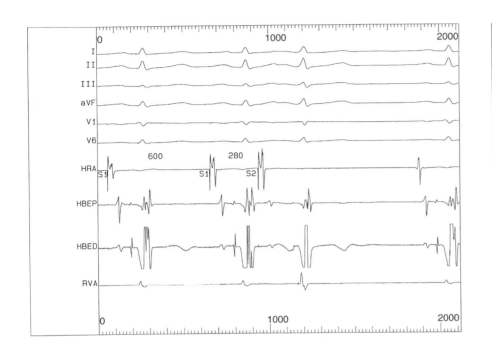
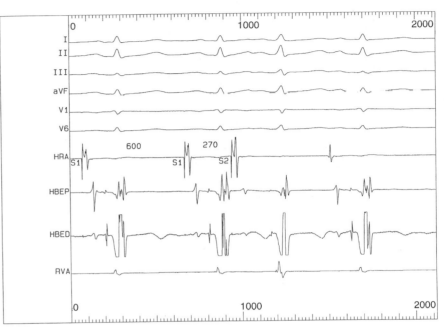

Figures 2–14A and 2–14B were recorded during right atrial pacing at CL 600 ms with a premature atrial complex of 280 ms (Fig. 2–14A) and 270 ms (Fig. 2–14B). What is the most likely cause of the difference in sinus return cycle after the premature complex?

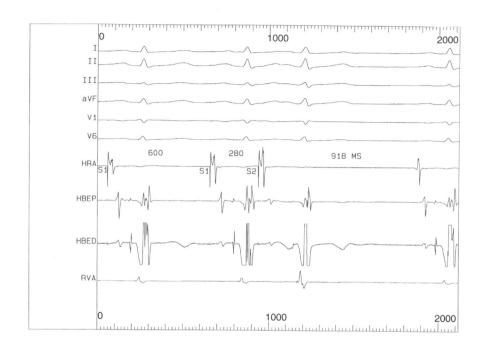

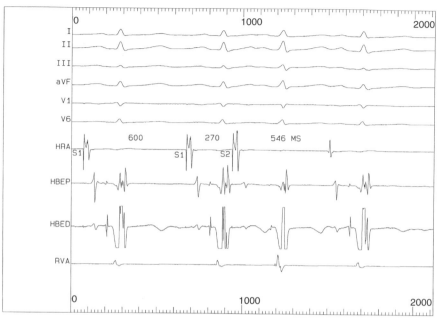

## Explanation:

In Fig. 2–14C, a PAC conducts to the ventricle and the subsequent sinus complex occurs 918 ms later. In Fig. 2–14D, a more premature atrial complex results in a sudden shortening of the return SCL to 546 ms. This may represent a sinus nodal echo or the attainment of the sinus node effective refractory period. In the latter case the PAC presumably did not invade the sinus node. Therefore, it was not reset allowing an earlier sinus complex to occur. This is one measure of sinus nodal function.

# Figure 2–15A

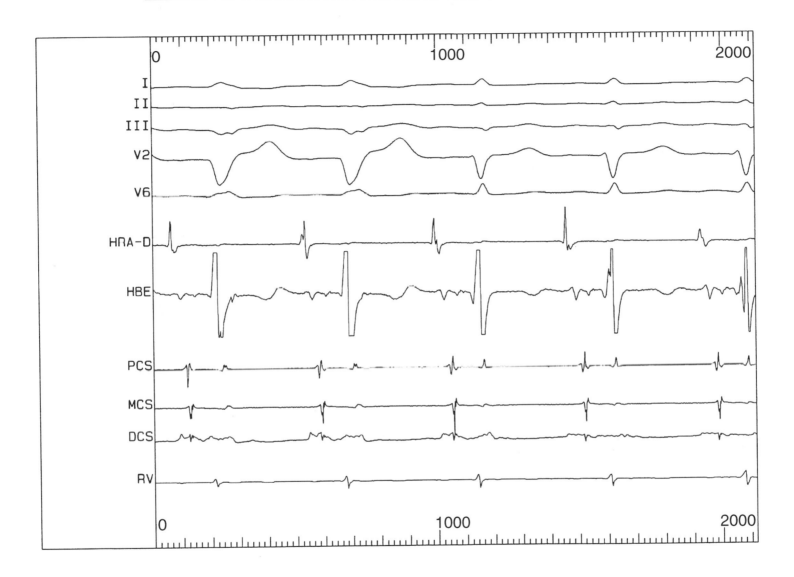

This recording was made during an electrophysiologic study in a
patient with an AP who just underwent radiofrequency catheter
ablation. What EP phenomena are present?

## Figure 2-15B

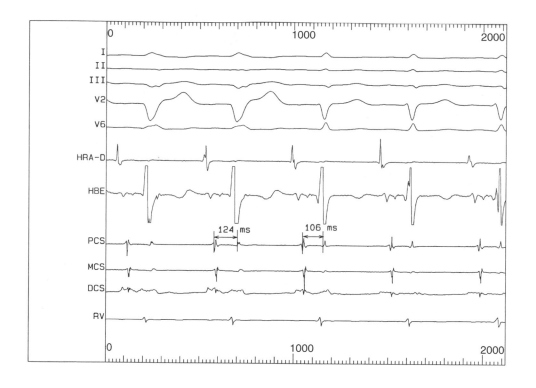

## Explanation:

This patient had a posterolateral AP with bidirectional conduction. Radiofrequency energy successfully ablated the AP. Shortly thereafter the patient was noted to have wide QRS complexes followed by narrow QRS complexes during sinus rhythm. The first two complexes represent LBBB aberrancy and not AP conduction. Note that the HV interval is similar for the narrow and wide QRS complexes. It is not clear why this patient had LBBB aberrancy at this part of the study, but he did have LBBB aberrancy during orthodromic AV reentry. Importantly, there is a definite change in the local AV interval recorded on the coronary sinus catheter. Note on the proximal coronary sinus electrogram the local AV interval is 124 ms during LBBB conduction and this becomes shorter (106 ms) during normal conduction. Since the activation time from the sinus node to the local atrial electrogram at the coronary sinus electrode remains constant (HRA-D to PCS), the difference in local conduction time results from delayed activation of the posterior left ventricular wall during LBBB.

In summary, the two key observations present are LBBB aberrancy and its accompanying effect to delay conduction to the left ventricular posterior wall.

## *Figure 2–16A*

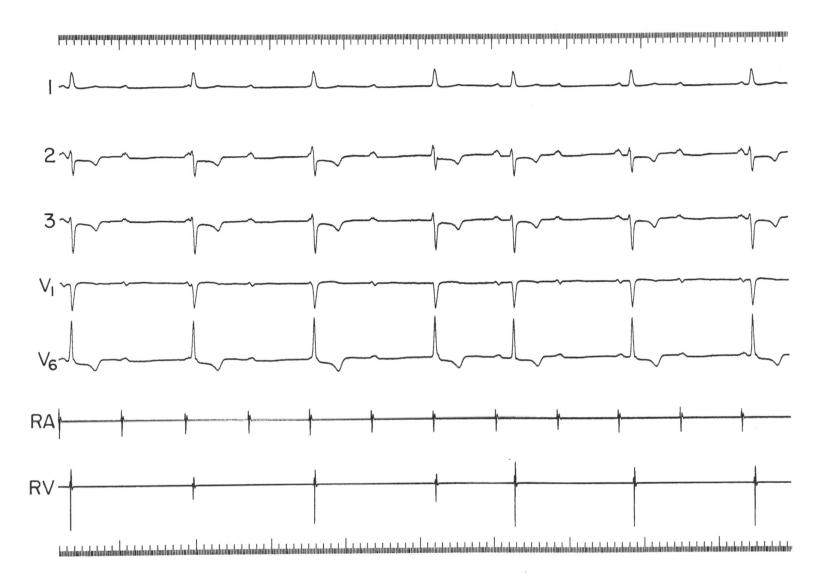

This 62-year-old man underwent radiofrequency ablation of the AV
node 30 min prior to this record. Is this complete AV block?

# Figure 2–16B

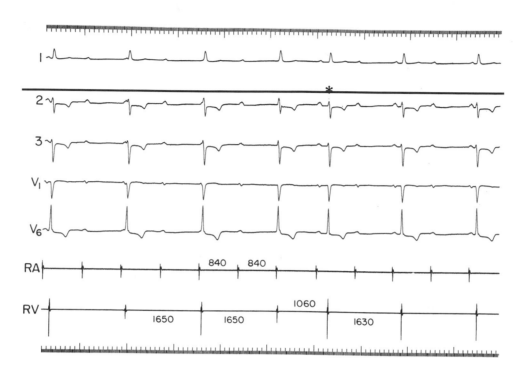

## Explanation:

The atrial CL is 840 ms and the ventricular CL is 1650 ms. The QRS has normal supraventricular morphology, compatible with a junctional escape rhythm. AV block appears to be complete except for the occasional ventricular cycle that is premature (*asterisk*). The cycle *after* the premature beat is "on time," indicating that the junctional pacemaker has been reset. This capture beat always occurred if the P wave was coupled to the previous QRS by a critical interval (RP > 870 ms will capture) and the pattern observed on the figure was repetitive. AV block is obviously not "complete" although it may be described as high grade. The conducted P wave has a PR interval of 220 ms, the minimal time needed to capture the junctional focus. A P wave occurring less than 220 ms from the subsequent QRS will have no chance to capture the ventricles.

# Figure 2–17A

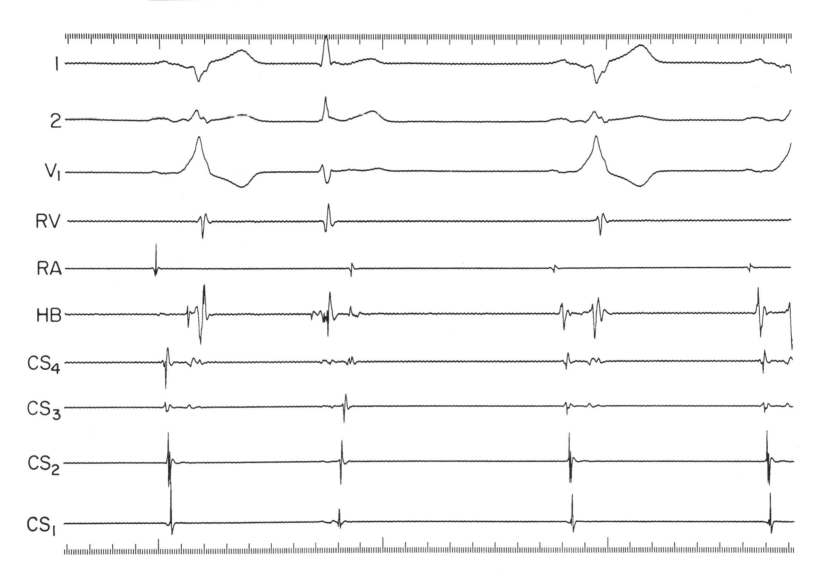

This patient with the WPW pattern presented clinically with a regular, wide QRS tachycardia. Based on the data in this figure, is this likely to be antidromic tachycardia?

## Figure 2–17B

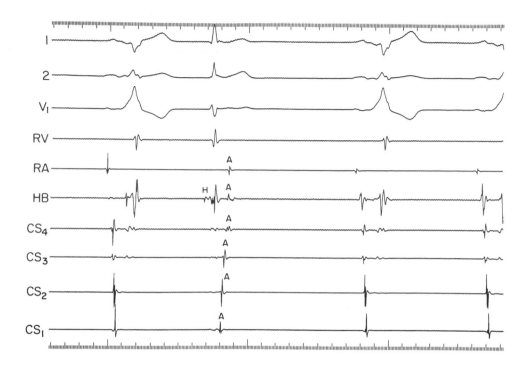

**Explanation:**

The first cycle is sinus cycle and is preexcited with onset of QRS preceding the His deflection. The second cycle, a His extrasystole, is preceded by a His deflection and the QRS has normalized. His extrasystoles are usually observed during or shortly after positioning of the His bundle catheter. In this instance, retrograde conduction to the atrium is occurring over a left lateral AP as evidenced by earliest atrial activation at the distal coronary sinus ($CS_1$). There is no evidence for retrograde conduction over the AV node, a condition that must be possible to enable antidromic tachycardia, a tachycardia circuit with anterograde conduction over the AP, and retrograde conduction over AV node. However, retrograde conduction over the AV node may have a longer conduction time than the AP and could become apparent only after retrograde block over the AP. Furthermore, retrograde conduction over the AV node could be catecholamine dependent. Consequently, antidromic tachycardia as a clinical tachycardia is unlikely but not precluded by this record.

## *Figure 2–18A*

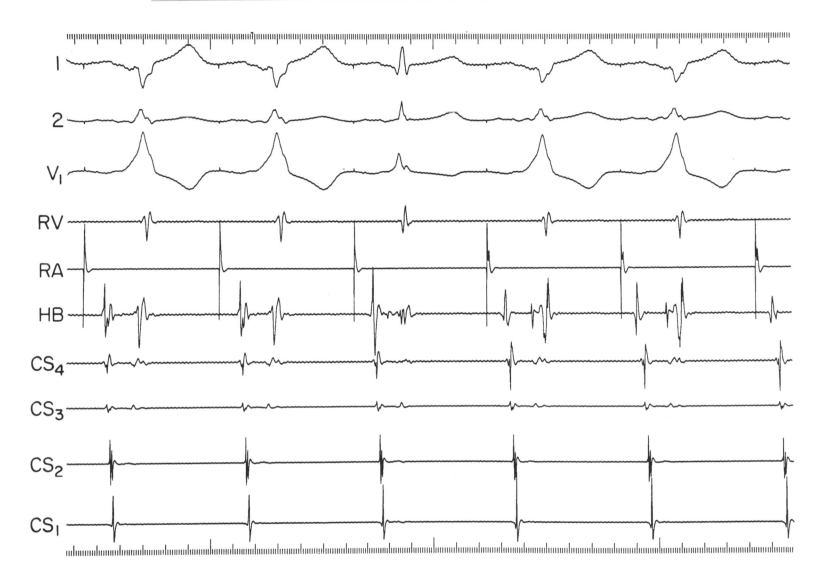

Same patient as in Figure 2–17. Why has the QRS apparently normalized?

# *Figure 2–18B*

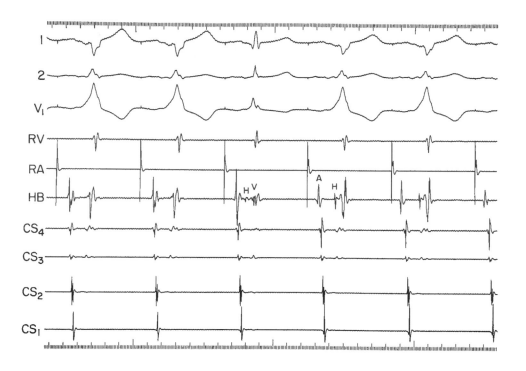

## Explanation:

Normalization of the preexcited QRS in this instance could theoretically occur (1) after block over the AP, (2) with the fortuitous occurrence of a PVC after atrial activation (pseudonormalization), or (3) with the fortuitous occurrence of a His extrasystole, resulting in more activation of the ventricle over the normal conduction system than the AP. The continued presence of preexcitation, albeit less marked, and the apparent shortening of the AH interval favors the diagnosis of a fortuitous His extrasystole, resulting in a more normal appearance of the QRS.

# *Figure 2–19A*

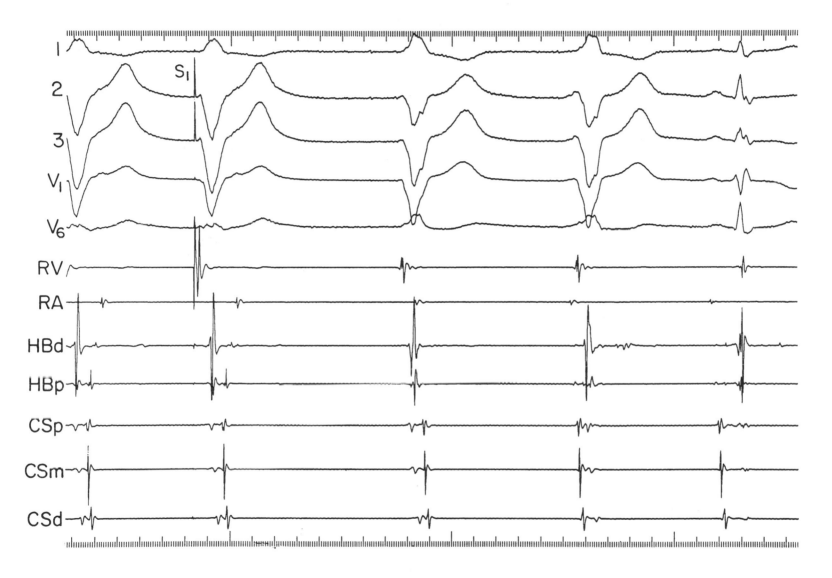

This patient had a right AV pathway with a long conduction time. After cessation of pacing, two cycles with QRS identical to the preexcited QRS are observed consistently. How is this explained?

# Figure 2–19B

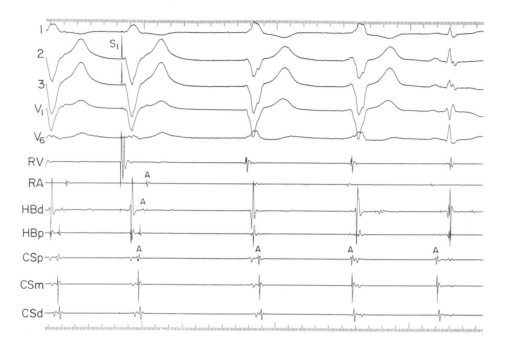

## Explanation:

The relative sinus pauses after cessation of pacing allowed the emergence of automaticity in this right-sided pathway. APs may exhibit intrinsic automaticity, especially those with decremental properties and long conduction times. The two cycles could theoretically be ventricular in origin but the QRS morphology identical to the preexcited QRS argues against this.

# Figure 2–20A

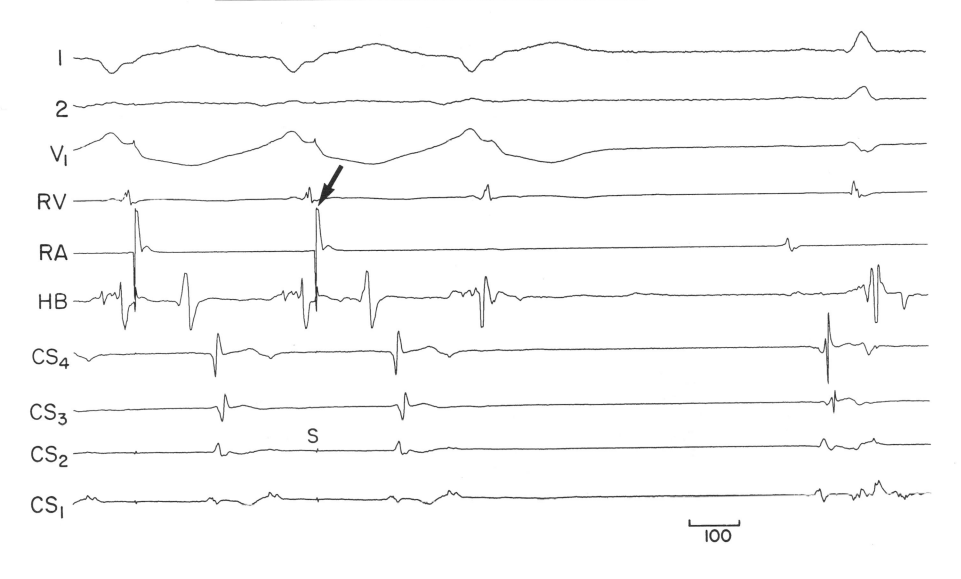

This patient's preexcitation pattern was not evident on the surface ECG in the absence of atrial pacing at a rapid rate. Why not?

# Figure 2-20B

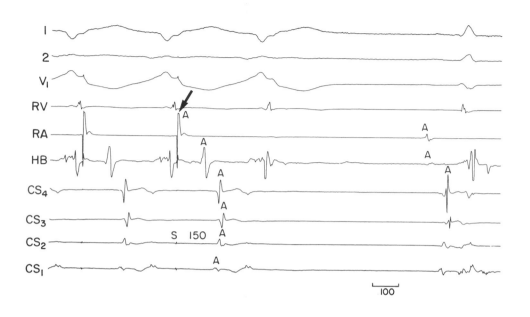

**Explanation:**

The QRS morphology during pacing clearly shows a left lateral preexcitation pattern. The record also reveals impressive intra-atrial and interatrial conduction delay during pacing (S to A interval is 150 ms). In sinus rhythm, this delay contributes to the relatively lesser contribution of the left AP to ventricular activation. In sinus rhythm, the atrium at the His bundle electrode (HB) is activated approximately 20 ms after the right atrial site (RA), whereas the atrial electrogram near the AP insertion site in the distal coronary sinus (CS₂) is only activated 60 ms later. The latter allows more direct imput into the AV node than the left AP, causing the balance of fusion to be shifted to the normal conducting system. Importantly, pacing prolongs AV node conduction time but not AP conduction time.

# Figure 2-21A

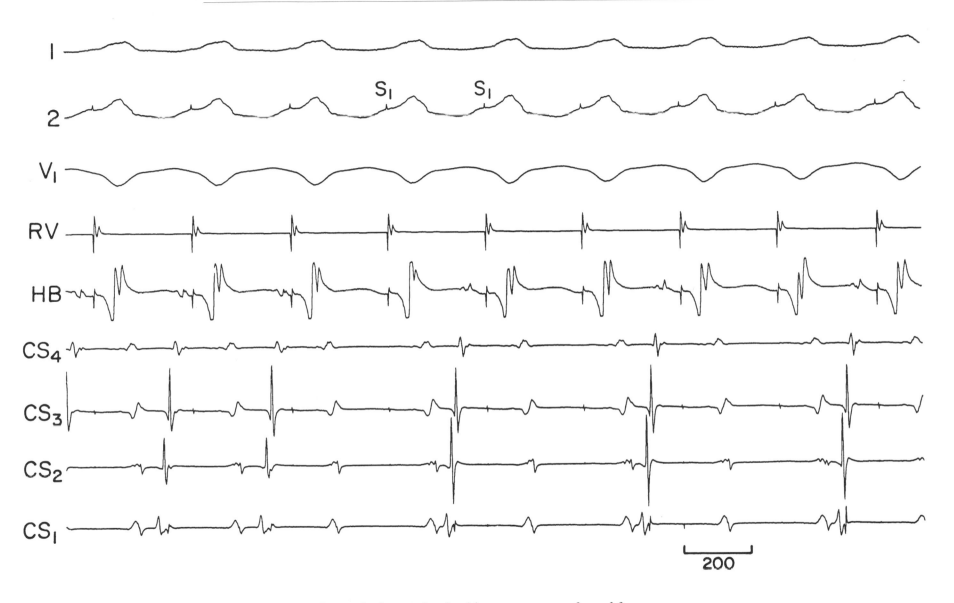

Incremental ventricular pacing in this young man referred for recurrent SVT revealed this phenomenon. How many APs are present?

# *Figure 2–21B*

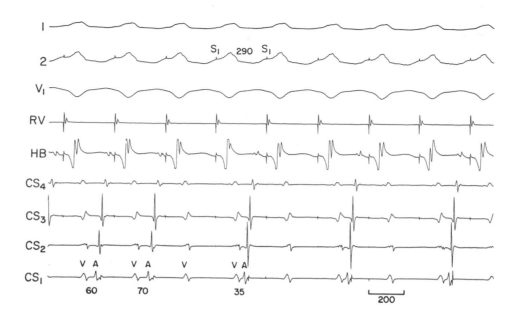

## Explanation:

Incremental ventricular pacing has resulted in retrograde block. Earliest retrograde atrial activation is occurring in the distal coronary sinus ($CS_1$) compatible with conduction over a left lateral AP. The interesting observation is the prolongation of the local VA interval prior to block with subsequent *shortening* of the VA interval in the first ventricular cycle after the blocked one. APs in general conduct in an "all or none" fashion and Wenckebach type block is unusual. *Decremental* conduction such as this, however, is occasionally observed in patients with APs. The retrograde atrial activation sequence appears similar regardless of the VA interval. It is generally believed that this decremental conduction is related to the intrinsic properties of a given AP although it is conceivable that there are multiple, closely spaced APs with different VA intervals.

## Figure 2–22A

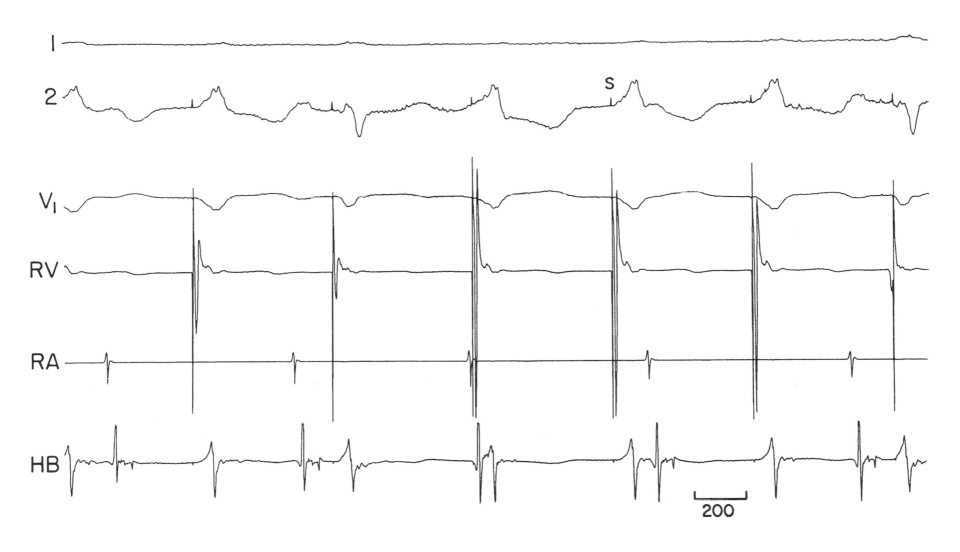

The tracing shows ventricular pacing. Does this patient need a pacemaker?

# *Figure 2–22B*

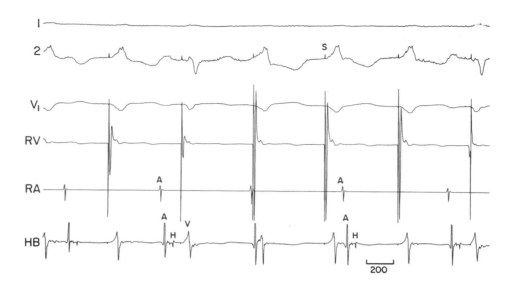

## Explanation:

The tracing demonstrates ventriculoatrial dissociation. The atrial activation sequence is high to low, beginning at the right atrial electrogram. The third complex is a *capture-fusion* beat, demonstrating fusion between the ventricular paced cycle and the sinus cycle. The seventh complex appears to be a pure capture beat as the pacing stimulus artifact occurs too late to capture the ventricle. AV block in this situation is physiologic and is best explained by concealed retrograde conduction of the paced ventricular rhythm into the normal AV conduction system. The level of block is below the recorded His bundle. Block below the recorded His is generally pathologic but can be accounted for in this case by concealed retrograde conduction. The patient was undergoing study for suspected tachycardia and was otherwise asymptomatic. He does not need a pacemaker based solely on the EP observations.

# Figure 2–23A

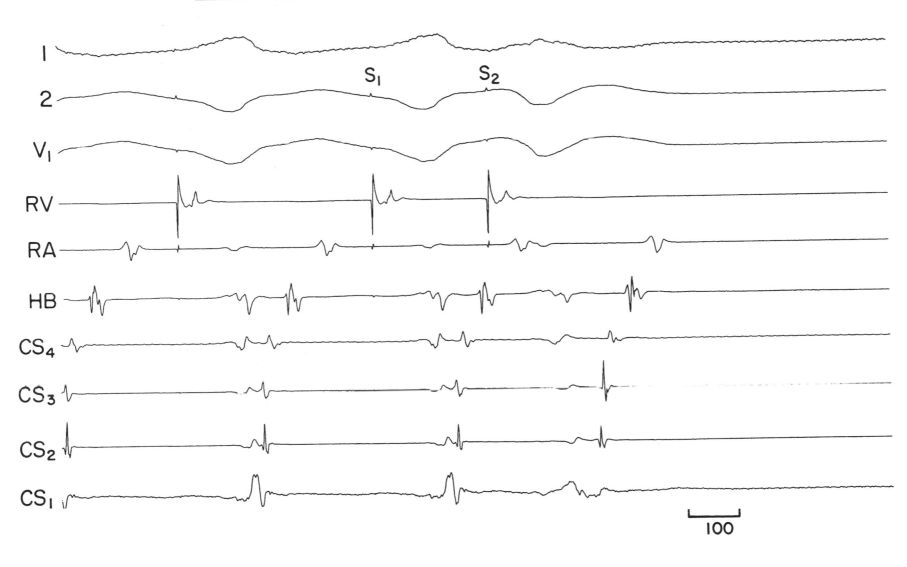

This patient was referred for AP ablation. Ventricular extrastimulus testing is displayed with the last two beats of the drive and the extrastimulus shown. CS₄ is at the orifice of the coronary sinus and CS₃ to CS₁ are progressively distal. How many APs are present?

# *Figure 2–23B*

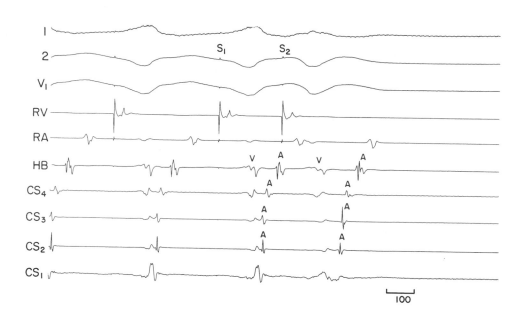

## Explanation:

The retrograde atrial activation sequence is eccentric, with earliest activation in the distal coronary sinus clearly indicating a left lateral AP. The VA interval prolongs abruptly with the extrastimulus. This may represent decremental conduction over the AP as illustrated in Figure 2–21. In this case, however, there is a subtle but distinct change in atrial activation sequence, which in this patient represented a second AP slightly more distal to the first with a longer VA conduction time. This was verified by ablation.

## Figure 2–24A

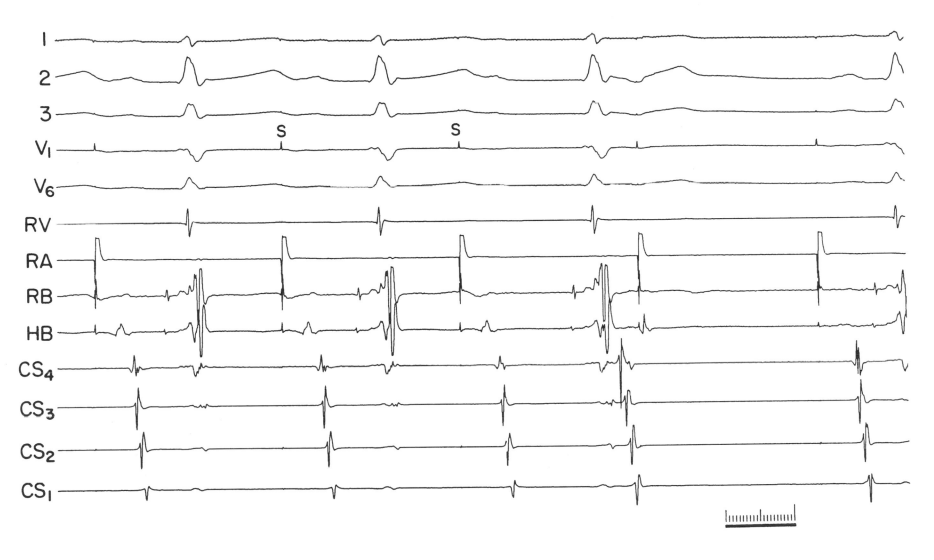

This tracing was observed during atrial pacing in a young patient studied for tachycardia. The interval between stimuli (S) is 520 ms. CS₄ is at the orifice of the coronary sinus and CS₃ to CS₁ are progressively distal. What should be ablated?

# Figure 2-24B

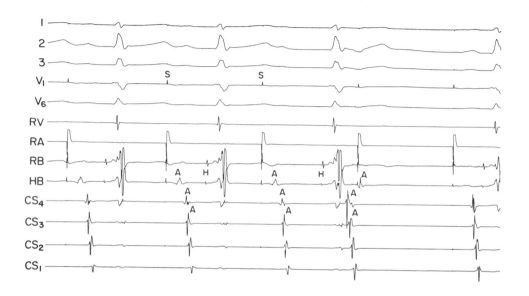

## Explanation:

During atrial pacing, there is a sudden prolongation of the AH interval, representing a shift to a slow AV node pathway (third QRS). This is associated with an atrial echo cycle that does not subsequently conduct to the ventricle. The atrial echo largely preempts the stimulus artifact (local atrial capture may be present but clearly does not depolarize most of the atrium), which is inscribed shortly thereafter. The atrial echo shows earliest activation just inside the orifice of the coronary sinus ($CS_4$). This is compatible with either conduction over a posteroseptal AP or a retrograde AV node pathway. In this particular study, observations during sustained tachycardia observed elsewhere verified the diagnosis of a posteroseptal AP. Atrial reciprocation in this patient required conduction delay, which in this instance was afforded by prolonged conduction over the slow AV node pathway. In this instance, slow pathway ablation could be reasonably contemplated to prevent tachycardia if ablation of the posteroseptal pathway was otherwise problematic.

## Figure 2-25A

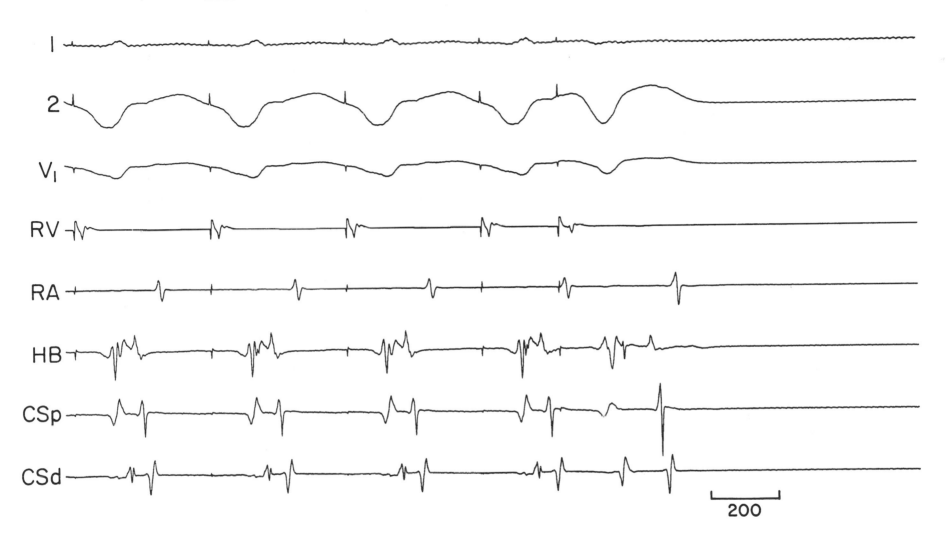

During progressively more rapid ("incremental") ventricular pacing in this patient, the VA conduction time changed only marginally from the slowest to the fastest paced rate prior to block. With ventricular extrastimulus testing, however, there was sudden prolongation of the VA interval. Why?

*Figure 2–25B*

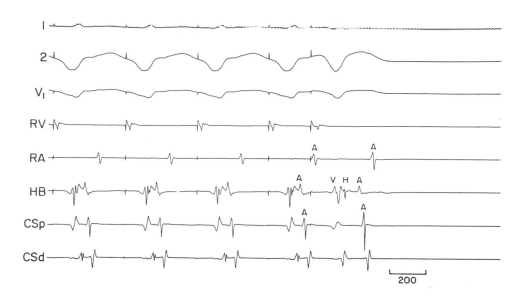

**Explanation:**

The His deflection is not obvious during the ventricular drive but clearly emerges after ventricular depolarization subsequent to the extrastimulus. The abrupt change in CL results in conduction delay in the HPS, which is usually not observed during incremental ventricular pacing with a more gradual decrement in CL. A sudden "jump" of the VA interval with ventricular extrastimulus testing is usually related to prolongation of the VH interval rather than being representative of dual AV node pathways. It is not unusual to observe only minimal changes in the VA interval during incremental ventricular pacing, an observation that does not necessarily suggest the presence of an AP.

# Figure 2–26A

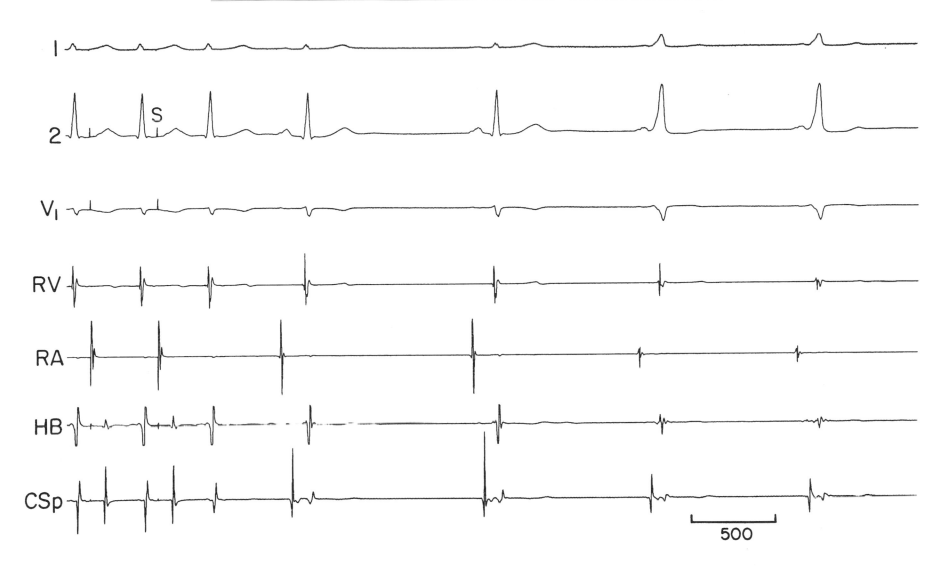

This patient was referred for assessment of the Wolff-Parkinson-White syndrome. Preexcitation was observed during incremental atrial pacing down to a CL of 400 ms at which point the QRS abruptly normalized. The end of this pacing run is illustrated in the figure. What phenomenon is observed?

## *Figure 2–26B*

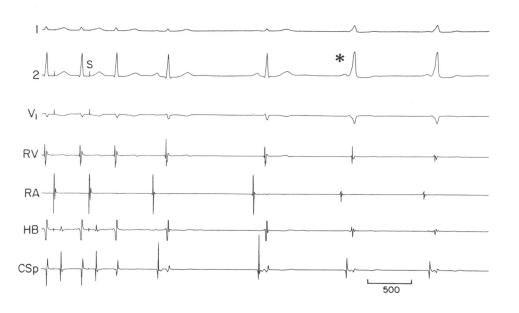

**Explanation:**

The QRS remains normal for the first two spontaneous sinus cycles after cessation of pacing. It is only the third spontaneous sinus cycle that results in resumption of preexcitation. Knowing that preexcitation persisted until CL 410 ms during incremental pacing would lead one to predict that the first two spontaneous cycles after termination of pacing should be preexcited since sufficient delay was present to permit recovery of excitability over the pathway. "Fatigue" is defined as a transient failure of conduction after repetitive excitation and was observed in this patient after the cessation of rapid pacing or a sufficiently premature extrastimulus. The duration of fatigue was dependent on both the rate and duration of pacing. Repetitive excitation may produce prolonged and persistent depolarization of the diastolic membrane potential, which is unfavorable to impulse propagation. The mechanism of this phenomenon is unknown.

## Figure 2–27A

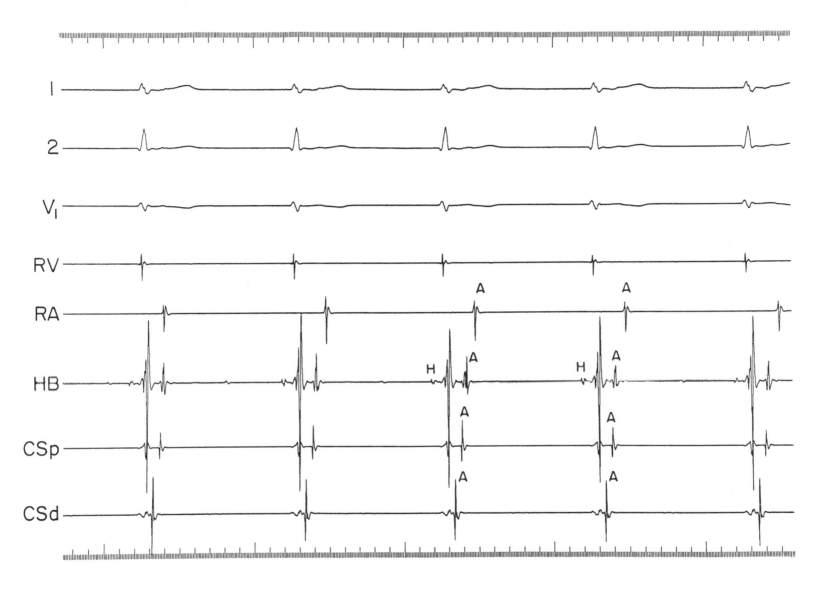

What is the differential diagnoses of this rhythm? How would one prove the diagnosis?

# *Figure 2-27B*

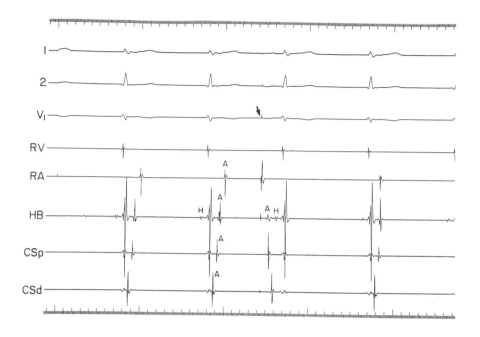

## Explanation:

The atrial activation sequence is eccentric (see Table 1–7) suggesting a diagnosis of atrial tachycardia or AV reentry. With either diagnosis, one must postulate the presence of a slow AV node pathway resulting in a very long AH interval. It is also noteworthy that the atrial activation pattern does not support the presence of a retrograde fast AV node pathway. Such a long AH interval (770 ms) would, however, be distinctly unusual for a beat conducted over the AV node.

A third possibility is a junctional rhythm with retrograde conduc-tion over a left lateral AP, the latter not directly involved in the mechanism of the rhythm. This third possibility does not require a slow pathway as part of the explanation. A premature atrial depolar-ization inserted in middiastole should and did clarify this diagnosis. It conducted with a short AH interval, verifying the diagnosis of junctional rhythm with retrograde conduction over an AP. If the long diastolic interval were occupied by slow pathway conduction, this atrial extrastimulus likely would not have conducted to the His and certainly not with a short AH interval.

# Chapter 3
# Narrow QRS Tachycardia

# Figure 3–1A

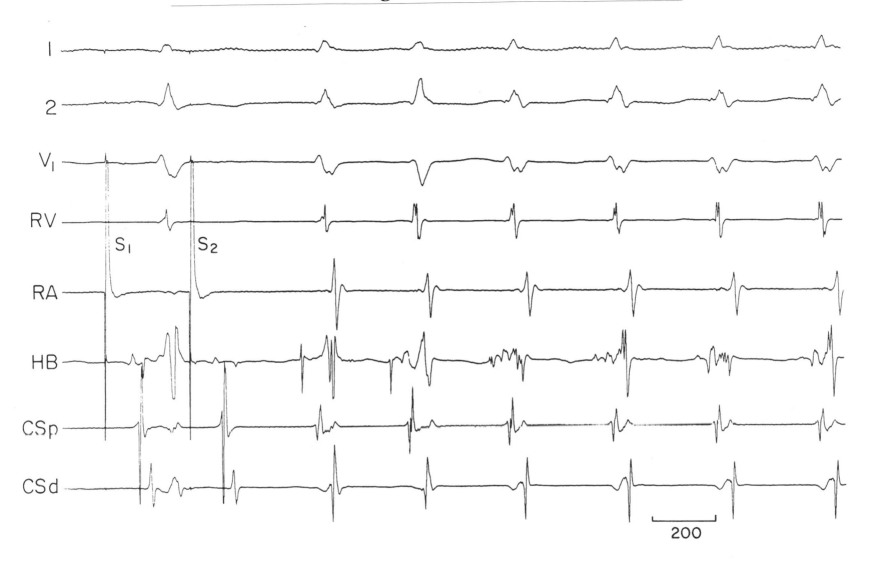

The patient is a young woman with paroxysmal tachycardia. Tachycardia is initiated by a critically timed atrial extrastimulus. What is the differential diagnosis and probable mechanism of the tachycardia?

*Figure 3–1B*

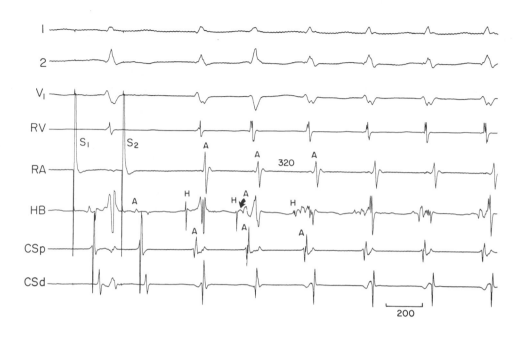

## Explanation:

The differential diagnosis of a narrow QRS tachycardia is presented in Chapter 1, Table 1–5. The tachycardia has a normal QRS, a cycle length of 320 ms, and a 1:1 AV relationship. The atrial activation is central with earliest activation at the His (*arrow*) where atrial activation precedes ventricular activation. This excludes sinus node reentry. The short VA interval rules out AV reentry. Although atrial tachycardia is not excluded, the apparent requirement of AH prolongation at the onset of tachycardia makes AV node reentry most likely. Maneuvers to assess AV node participation in tachycardia such as carotid sinus massage will confirm the diagnosis.

*Figure 3–2A*

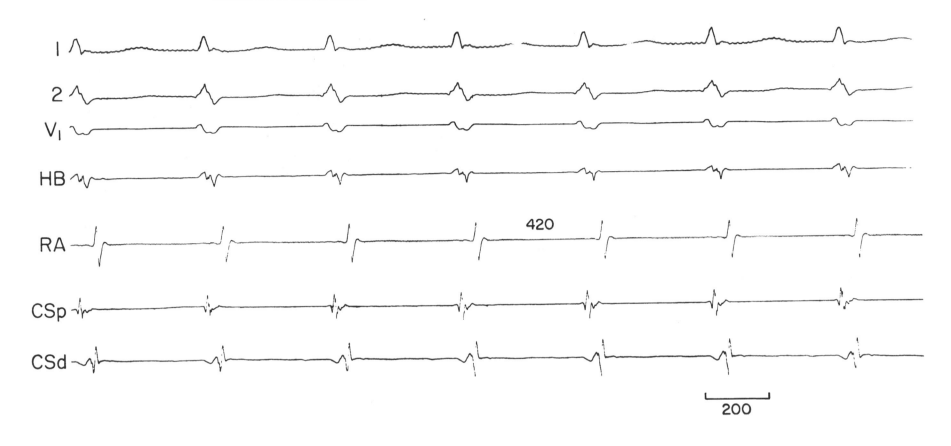

I

2

V$_1$

HB

RA                                          420

CSp

CSd

200

Same patient as in Fig. 3–1. There has been a sudden increase in the tachycardia cycle length to 420 ms (transition not recorded, His catheter out of position). What is the mechanism?

# Figure 3–2B

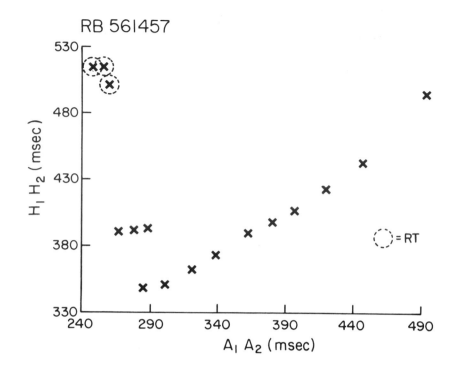

RB 561457

**Explanation:**

The new tachycardia appears identical to the original with the exception of the cycle length, which is longer entirely due to presumed prolongation of the AH interval. The His catheter is out of position but the absence of bundle branch block makes HV delay very unlikely. The most probable mechanism is AV node reentry using a second "slower" slow AV node pathway. The presence of two tachycardia rates could have been predicted by examination of the curve relating AV node conduction time ($H_1 H_2$) to prematurity of an atrial extrastimulus ($A_1 A_2$). This shows a double discontinuity, suggesting the existence of two slow pathways. RT signifies onset of tachycardia.

## Figure 3–3A

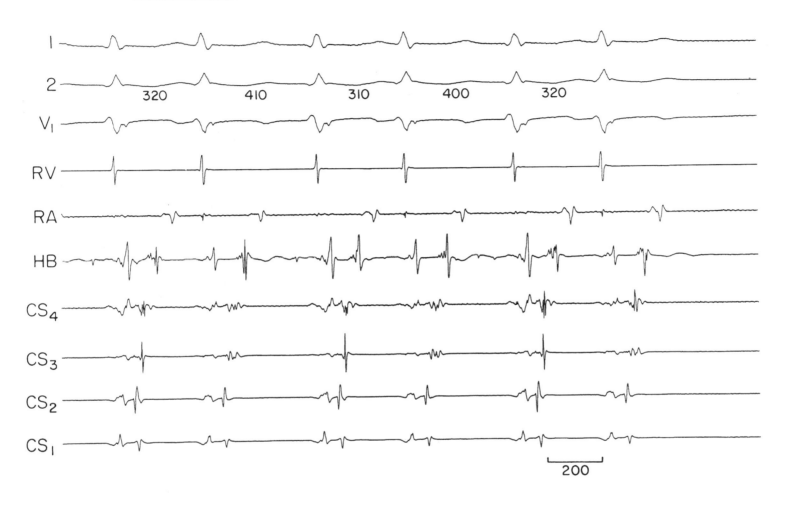

The record is from a young man with paroxysmal tachycardia. Tachycardia was never recorded because it always stopped prior to his arrival in the emergency department. The 12-lead ECG was normal. Induction of tachycardia was by atrial extrastimuli and required critical AH prolongation. Why did his tachycardia always stop spontaneously? $CS_4$ to $CS_1$ are coronary sinus electrograms from proximal (4) to distal (1), respectively. $CS_4$ is positioned near the orifice of the coronary sinus.

# Figure 3–3B

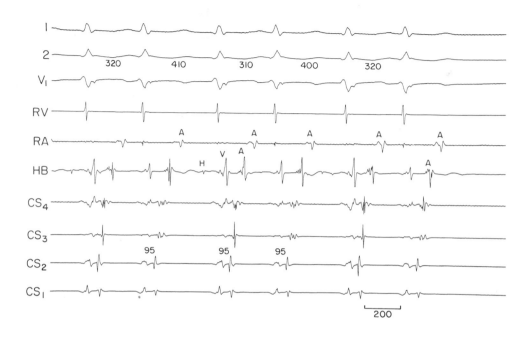

## Explanation:

The tachycardia is irregular and the cycle length alternates from approximately 300 to 400 ms due entirely to change in the AH interval. This suggests anterograde conduction over dual AV node pathways and dual pathway physiology was indeed observed during atrial extrastimulus testing. The atrial activation is eccentric (distal CS first), suggesting left atrial tachycardia or AV reentry over a left lateral AP. AV reentry was verified during the study but could have been deduced by two observations. Spontaneous termination occurred with an A, an unlikely event with atrial tachycardia because coincidental block in the AV node at the same time would have to be postulated. During oscillation of the cycle length, the change in AH precedes and predicts subsequent AA intervals, strongly implicating AV node participation. The oscillation in AV node conduction time facilitated spontaneous termination as fast pathway conduction impinged on the refractory period of the slow pathway.

Did this patient also have "typical" AV node reentry? It would not be expected (and was not observed) since slow pathway conduction during tachycardia did not result in retrograde fast AV node pathway conduction that would have preempted retrograde AP conduction.

## Figure 3–4A

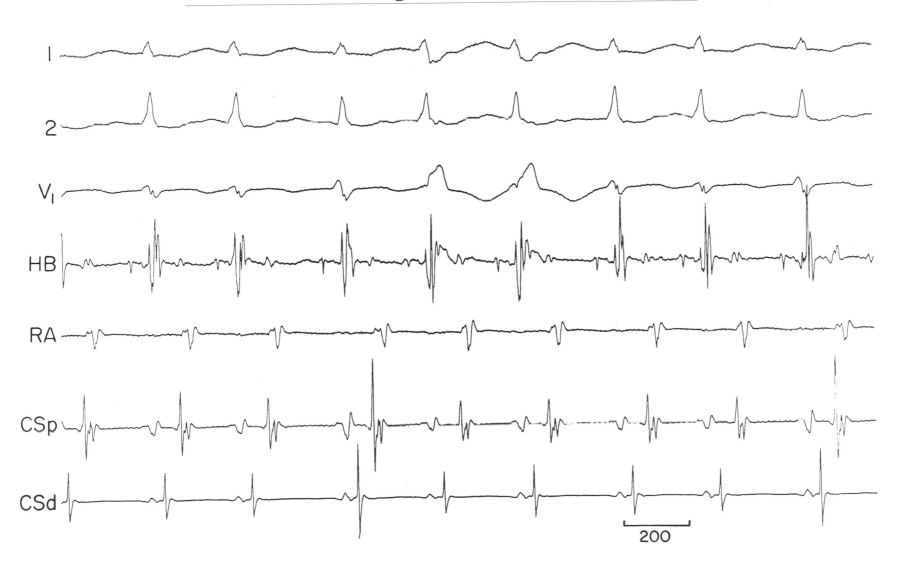

I

2

V₁

HB

RA

CSp

CSd

200

The record is from a young man otherwise well except for paroxysmal tachycardia. The surface ECG was normal. Tachycardia was induced with critically timed atrial extrastimuli. What is the mechanism, and why is there a change in the QRS morphology?

## *Figure 3–4B*

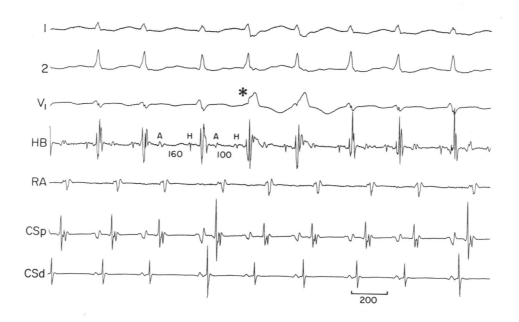

**Explanation:**

The tachycardia is irregular and this is related to two populations of AH intervals, approximately 100 and 160 ms. The atrial activation sequence is eccentric and the earliest A is recorded in the distal coronary sinus ($CS_d$). The differential diagnosis includes atrial tachy-cardia or AV reentry utilizing a left lateral AP. Atrial tachycardia is ruled out by the delay in atrial timing after a long AH, a fact suggesting that atrial activation is dependent on preceding AV conduction time (the VA interval is constant despite rate irregularity). RBBB aberration is observed after a long–short cycle sequence (Ashman phenomenon) related to AH changes.

## Figure 3–5A

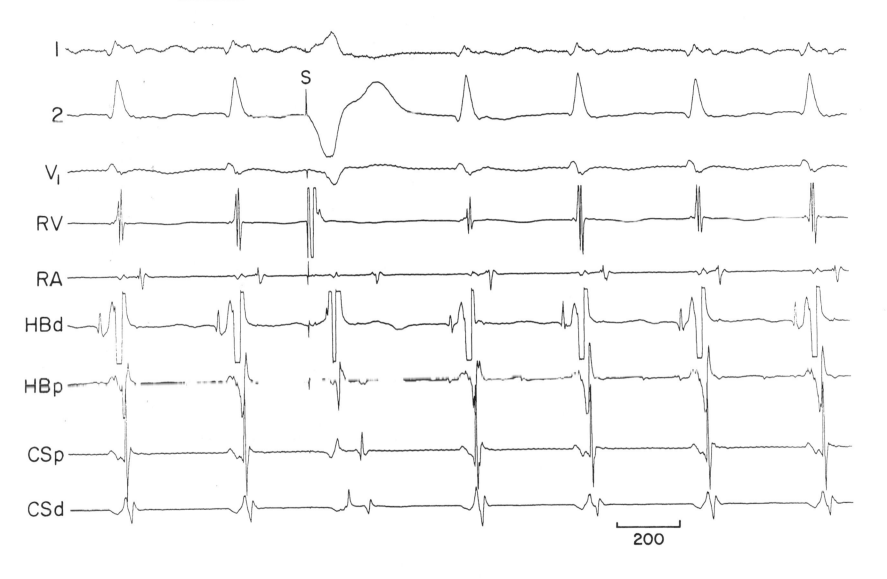

The PVC (*S*) programmed into the cardiac cycle during this regular
tachycardia proves the diagnosis of AV node reentry, doesn't it?

# Figure 3–5B

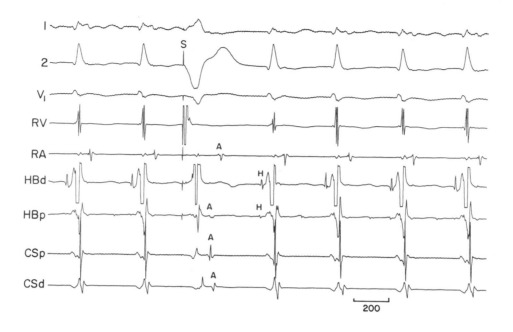

**Explanation:**

The tachycardia is regular. Both the long AH and the short VA interval support the diagnosis of AV node reentry and the atrial activation sequence is concentric as made clear by the early coupled PVC that advances the V and exposes the atrial electrograms. The PVC does not preexcite the next A and further supports the diagno-sis. However, failure to advance the A does *not* rule out atrial tachy-cardia. Indeed, failure to advance the A doesn't rule out atrioventric-ular reentry because the AP may be decremental or far away from a right ventricular extrastimulus (i.e., left lateral). In the present example, AV reentry is ruled out by the coincidental atrial and ventricular activation.

## *Figure 3–6A*

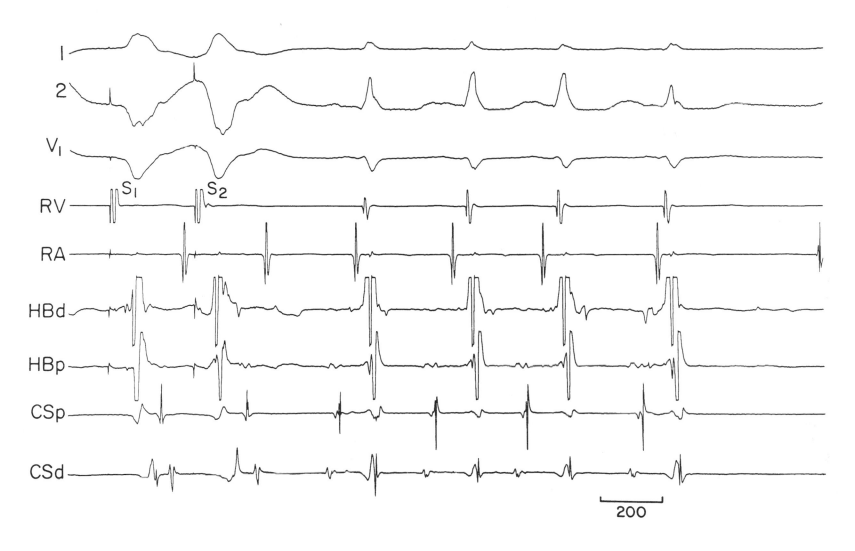

The patient was referred for assessment of supraventricular tachycardia, generally exercise induced. The following tachycardia was consistently induced by ventricular extrastimuli at a critical coupling interval as well as atrial extrastimuli. What is the mechanism of tachycardia?

# Figure 3-6B

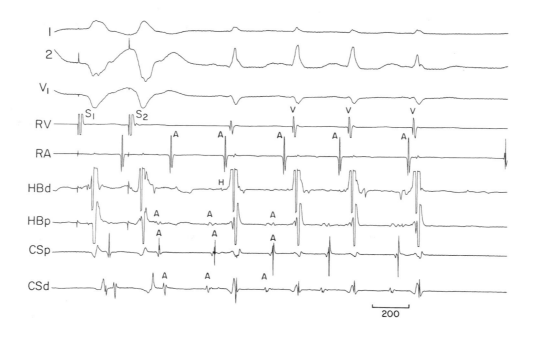

**Explanation:**

The ventricular extrastimulus conducts with a concentric atrial activation sequence with slight prolongation of the VA interval. This is compatible with conduction over the AV node. The next event is atrial activation with an eccentric atrial activation sequence with earliest atrial activation recorded at the distal coronary sinus electrogram ($CS_d$). Referring to Table 1–7, it is clear that this must be either an atrial tachycardia or AV reentry. The first spontaneous event in the tachycardia is atrial activation and points to the correct diagnosis of a left atrial tachycardia. A 2 : 1 phenomenon is remotely possible, that is, ventricular activation resulting from $S_2$ conducting to the atrium over both the AV node and a slowly conducting left lateral AP. This cannot be entirely ruled out from this record but is unlikely because of the variability of the apparent V to A interval during tachycardia.

## Figure 3-7A

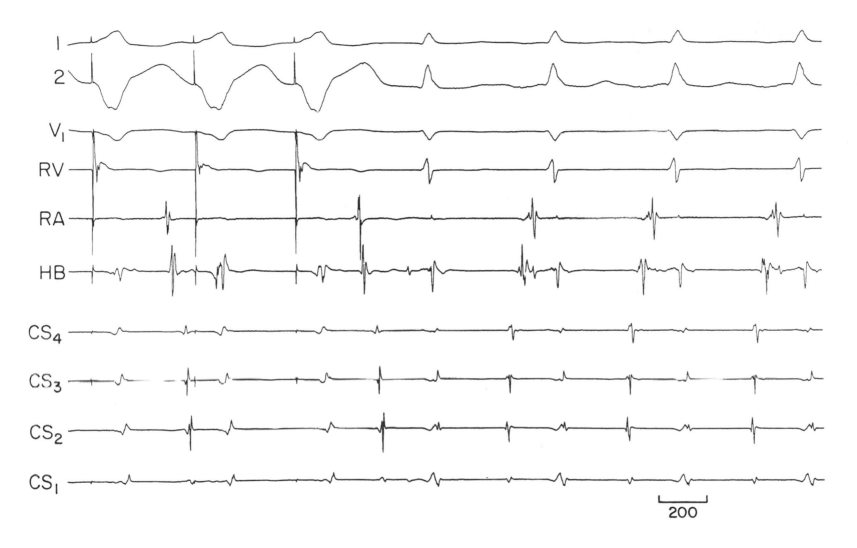

This tachycardia was initiated relatively reproducibly by a burst of ventricular pacing, as shown, with no apparent VA conduction during the burst. However, tachycardia only occurred if the first sinus com-plex after ventricular pacing conducted to the ventricle. What is the mechanism of tachycardia?

# Figure 3-7B

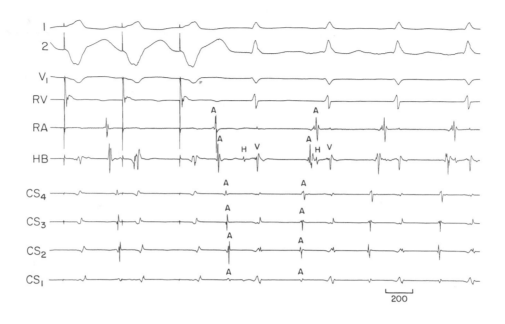

## Explanation:

The first atrial cycle after the last ventricular paced cycle has a high to low activation sequence and is sinus. This conducts with a relatively long AH interval, in all likelihood related to concealed retrograde conduction into the AV node by the last paced QRS. The first spontaneous tachycardia event is atrial activation with an eccentric activation sequence earliest at the distal coronary sinus (CS$_1$). The differential diagnosis then becomes (Table 1-7) atrial tachycardia or AV reentry over a left AP with a long conduction time. The latter is favored by the apparent requirement of previous AH prolongation as was observed during repetitive inductions. Tachycardia only occurred if the first sinus cycle after ventricular pacing conducted with AH prolongation. It was also known that eccentric retrograde atrial activation was observed with ventricular pacing at slower rates. However, atrial tachycardia could not be excluded from this record alone.

## Figure 3-8A

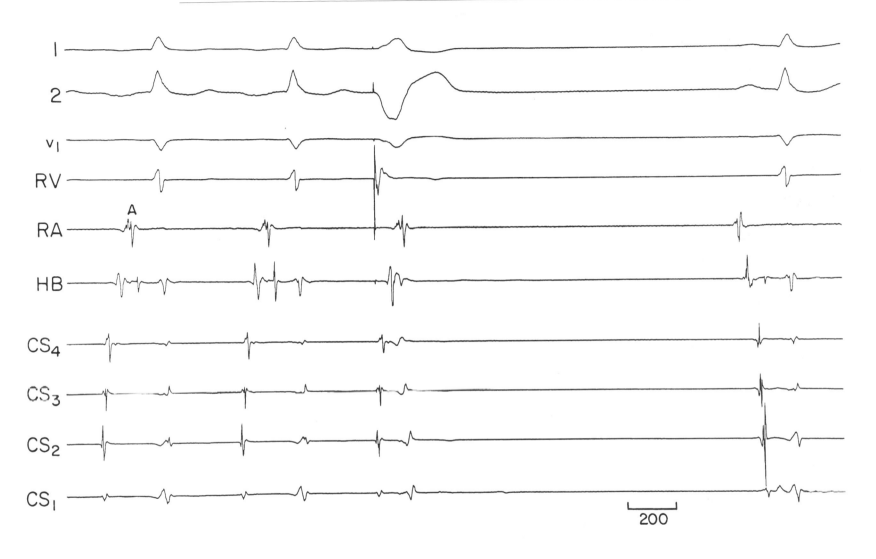

Data from the patient described in Fig. 3–7. A PVC programmed into the cardiac cycle at a critical coupling interval terminates tachycardia consistently. Does this clarify the mechanism?

# Figure 3–8B

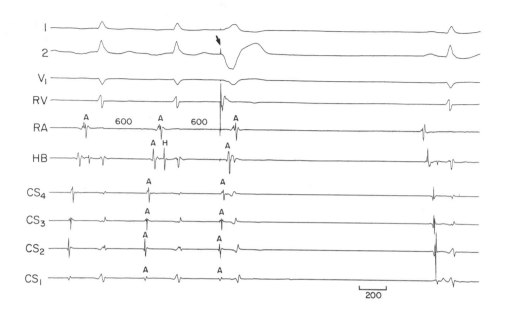

## Explanation:

This tachycardia was consistently terminated by a PVC that did not alter atrial activation or timing. This essentially excludes the diagnosis of atrial tachycardia, leaving the diagnosis of AV re-entry over a left lateral AP with a long conduction time, as was the case.

# Figure 3-9A

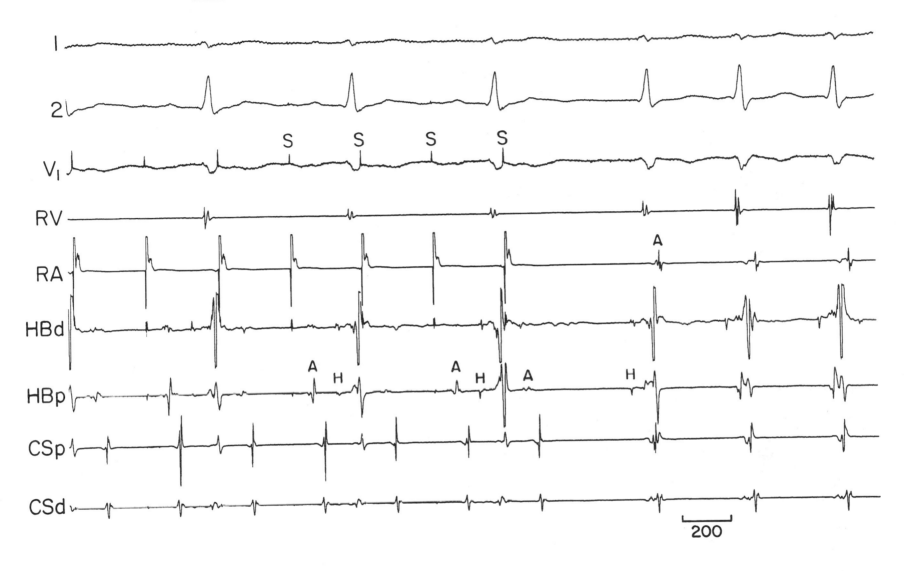

This tachycardia onset was recorded after termination of incremental atrial pacing that resulted in 2:1 AV block. What is the tachycardia mechanism and why did tachycardia start after termination of pacing?

# Figure 3–9B

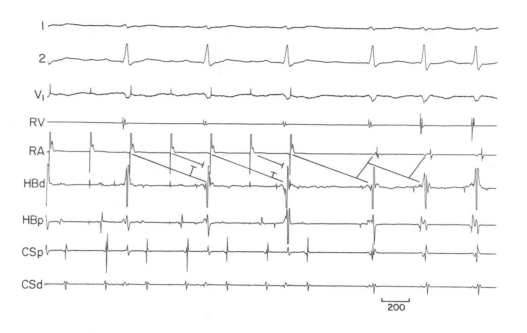

200

## Explanation:

The tachycardia mechanism is AV node reentry, as suggested by the extremely long AH at the onset, the concentric atrial activation sequence, and the simultaneous ventricular and atrial activation. Although atrial tachycardia or a junctional tachycardia (Table 1–6) could not be ruled out from this record, other criteria for AV node reentry were met during the study. During pacing, every second beat was conducted over the slow AV node pathway with manifest reentry aborted by the alternate atrial cycle that failed to conduct to the ventricle. With termination of pacing, slow pathway conduction is manifest and nothing prevents the return atrial cycle from continuing reentry. The excessive PR prolongation after the last paced atrial cycle is probably related to the effects of the previous nonconducted atrial cycle, which penetrated the slow pathway to some degree. The curve related $A_1–A_2$ to $A_H$ in this patient demonstrated a single but not a double discontinuity.

# Figure 3-10A

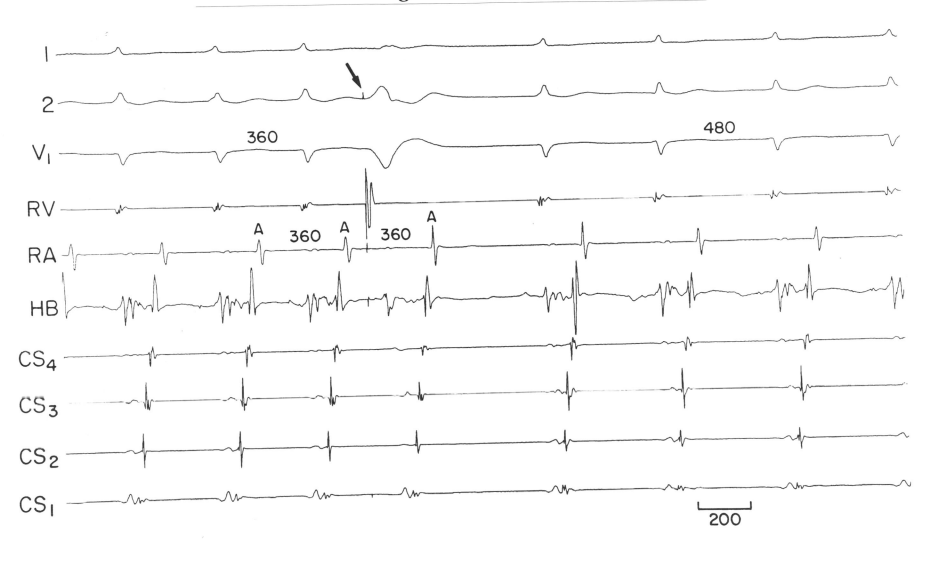

A PVC is introduced into this regular tachycardia at a relatively early coupling interval. It does not preexcite the atrium but changes the tachycardia. How does one explain this?

# Figure 3–10B

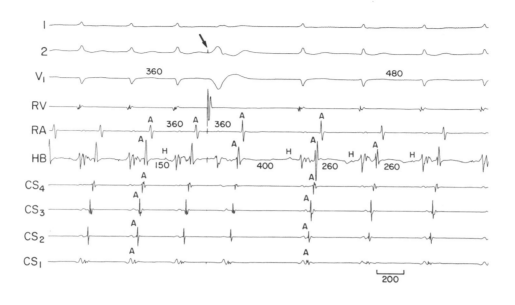

## Explanation:

The tachycardia is associated with an eccentric atrial activation sequence, leaving a differential diagnosis of atrial tachycardia or AV reentry over a left-sided AP. The PVC does not preexcite the atrium but prolongs the AH interval and converts the tachycardia to a slower one with a longer AH interval. Importantly, the change in atrial cycle length is linked to preceding change in the AH interval. Such an influence of a programmed PVC would be most unlikely with atrial tachycardia. It is probable that the PVC reached the AV node retrogradely, resulting in subsequent anterograde block of the fast pathway and subsequent conduction over the slow pathway. The first AH is prolonged more than the subsequent AH intervals, suggesting concealed conduction into the slow pathway by the PVC. This patient had AV reentry over a left lateral pathway with two distinct AH intervals consistent with dual AV node pathway physiology demonstrated by the atrial extrastimulus technique. Would one expect to have sustained AV node reentry induced in this patient? The absence of retrograde fast pathway conduction after the slow pathway is initially reached would suggest that the AV node reentrant circuit, at least under baseline conditions, is not operative.

# Figure 3-11A

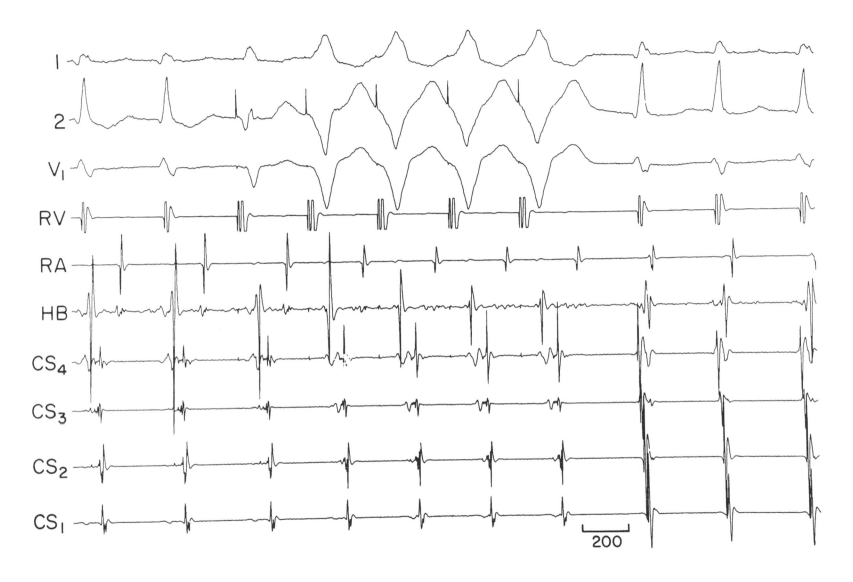

A brief burst of ventricular pacing is provided into this regular supraventricular tachycardia, resulting in change of activation sequence with minimal change in rate. What has happened?

## *Figure 3–11B*

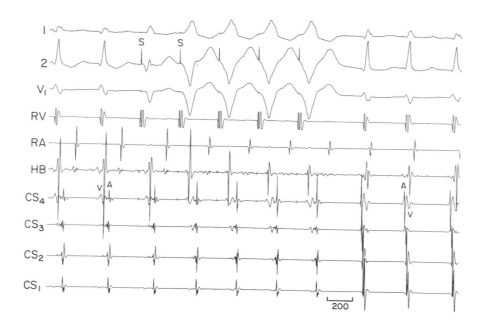

**Explanation:**

Two cycles of a regular SVT are shown at the beginning of the trace. The earliest atrial activation is in the proximal coronary sinus region ($CS_3$), approximately 10 to 20 mm from the orifice of the CS. The differential diagnosis at this point includes atrial tachycardia or AV reentry (Chapter 1, Table 1–7). Ventricular pacing results in entrainment of the tachycardia without change in the atrial activation sequence. Note that the second paced beat preexcites the atrium at a pacing interval that would not have been able to conduct retrogradely over the AV node. These two observations essentially confirm the diagnosis of atrioventricular reentry. After termination of pacing, a long AV interval is observed followed by a distinct change of atrial activation sequence. This tachycardia was subsequently confirmed to be AV node reentry. It is probable that entrainment of AV reentry by ventricular pacing resulted in concealed conduction into the AV node with block in the fast pathway after the first atrial cycle after cessation of pacing. Shift to the slow anterograde AV node pathway allowed reentrance up the fast AV nodal pathway with initiation of sustained AV node reentry. Where is the AP at this point? It is probable that there is concealed retrograde conduction into the AP that is preempted from capturing the atrium in whole or in part by retrograde activation over the fast AV node pathway.

# Figure 3–12A

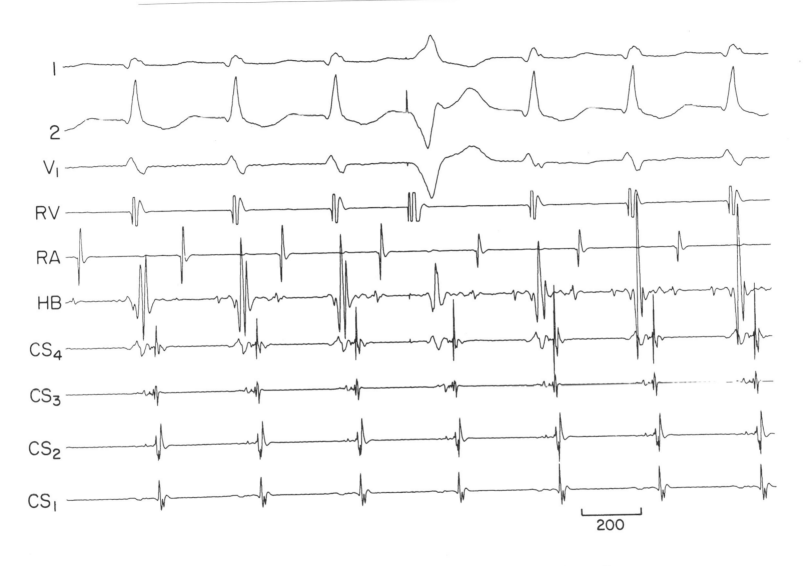

A PVC programmed into the cardiac cycle during the tachycardia
rules out AV reentry as the mechanism of tachycardia, does it not?

## Figure 3–12B

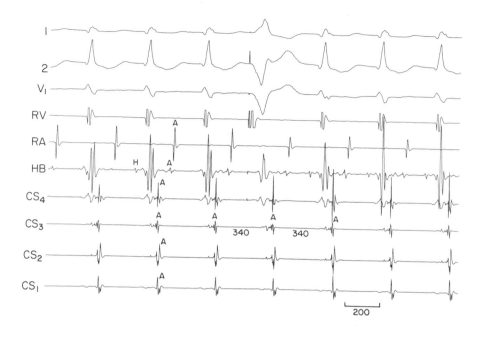

**Explanation:**

The earliest activation during this tachycardia occurs in the region of the orifice of the coronary sinus and left paraseptal area (CS$_4$, CS$_3$). The mechanism of this tachycardia could be AV reentry, atypical AV node reentry, or atrial tachycardia. A PVC delivered during His refractoriness that preexcites the subsequent atrial activation must be conducting over an AP. However, failure to preexcite (as is the case here) is not helpful and leaves the differential diagnosis open.

Failure of a PVC to preexcite during AV reentry may be related to distance of the stimulating catheter from the AP and the reentrant circuit. In the example shown, it would be useful to position the pacing catheter at the base of the heart near the site of the AP and repeat the programmed stimulation during tachycardia. This will invariably demonstrate preexcitation in AV reentry unless the AP exhibits "decremental" or rate-dependent conduction, which offsets the prematurity of the extrastimulus. This patient had AV reentry.

## Figure 3–13A

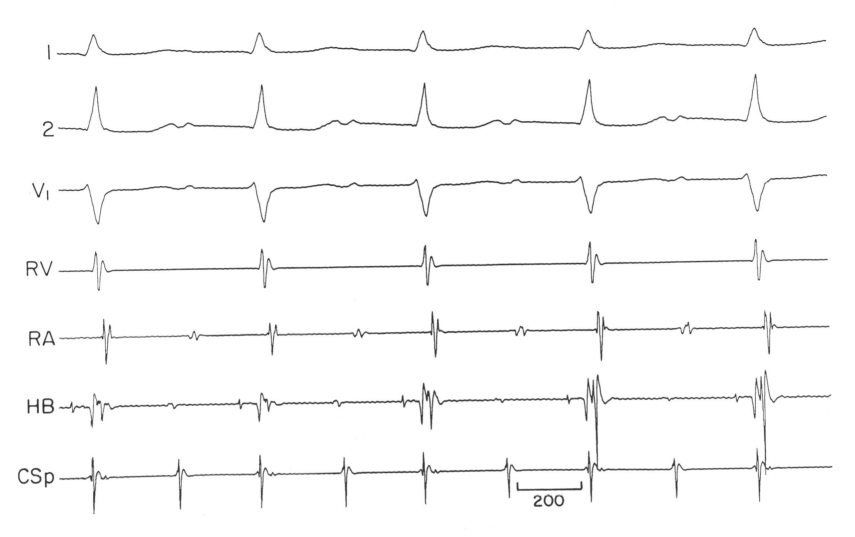

At EP testing, this patient with a history of SVT had regular SVT induced by an atrial extrastimulus that achieved a critical AH interval. The tachycardia was compatible with AV node reentry although the curve relating AH to prematurity of the atrial extrastimulus was continuous. A 2:1 AV block occurred spontaneously during this tachycardia and was recorded. What is the likely diagnosis?

# Figure 3–13B

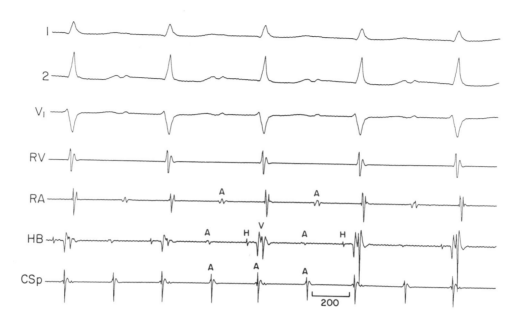

## Explanation:

The differential diagnosis is atrial tachycardia or AV node reentry. The distinction cannot be made definitively on examination of this tracing alone. However, note that the atrial electrogram of the blocked cycle is virtually at the midpoint between two QRS complexes, a feature favoring AV node reentry with 2:1 AV block. Another clue to AV node reentry is the characteristic narrow P wave during tachycardia compared with a longer duration during sinus rhythm. If there is AV node reentry with AV block, the block is occurring above the level of the recorded His. This also suggests that the final common pathway is also above the recorded His. However, the recorded His of conducted complexes has a low amplitude and it can be argued that failure to record the His deflection of nonconducted cycles is related to catheter position. Ablation in the slow pathway region eliminated all tachycardia.

# Figure 3–14A

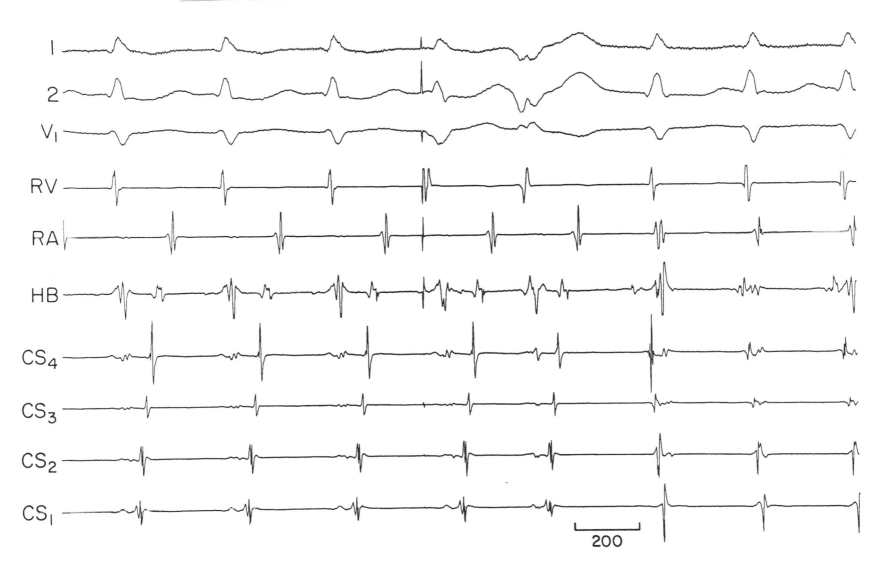

A PVC programmed into the cardiac cycle during this tachycardia resulted in a change in tachycardia cycle length. How does one explain the observations? Will ablation at a single site cure this patient?

3 NARROW QRS TACHYCARDIA

# Figure 3-14B

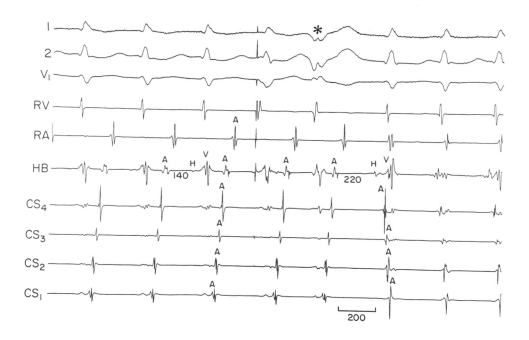

## Explanation:

At the onset, the tachycardia is associated with an eccentric atrial activation sequence (distal CS first). The differential diagnosis is atrial tachycardia versus AV reentry utilizing a left lateral AP as the retrograde limb of a circuit. A PVC introduced into the cycle at the time of His bundle refractoriness fails to affect the tachycardia circuit. However, a spontaneous PVC (*) occurs relatively earlier in the cycle and readily preexcites the atrium in the proportion to prematurity of the ventricular ectopic, supporting a diagnosis of AV reentry. The morphology of the spontaneous PVC suggests a left ventricular origin, explaining why the PVC preexcites the atrium over a left lateral pathway more readily than the induced one from the right ventricular apex. With preexcitation of the atrium (essentially a premature atrial complex), the subsequent AH interval prolongs suddenly, indicating block in the fast AV node pathway and shift to a slow AV node pathway. Subsequent retrograde fast AV node pathway activation then perpetuates sustained AV node reentry. This patient requires ablation of both the AP and the slow AV node pathway.

# Figure 3–15A

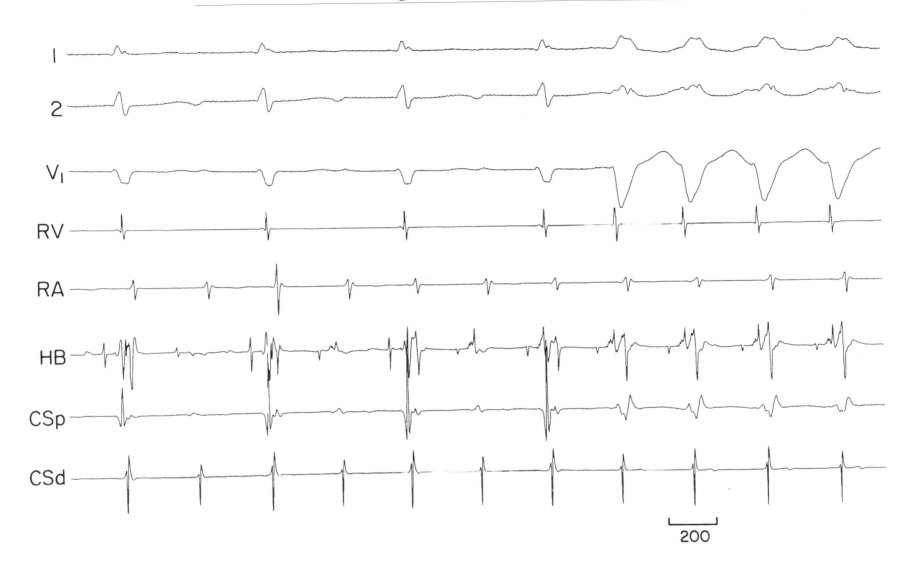

I

2

V₁

RV

RA

HB

CSp

CSd

200

This tachycardia was induced by a critically timed atrial extrastimulus associated with prolongation of the AH interval. What is the mechanism of tachycardia?

# Figure 3–15B

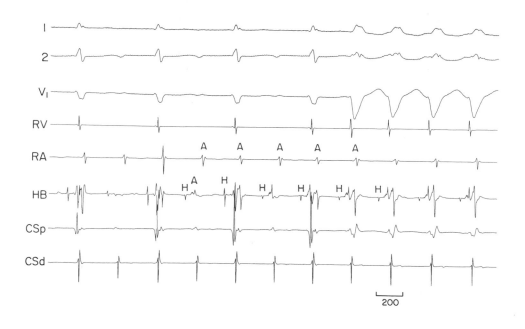

## Explanation:

The tracing begins with a supraventricular tachycardia with 2:1 AV block. The activation sequence is central with earliest recorded atrial activation at the His bundle electrogram. There is an abrupt transition to 1:1 AV conduction. Resumption of 1:1 conduction is associated with LBBB aberration, commonly noted in this situation. SVT with AV block immediately suggests atrial tachycardia as the mechanism. However, the apparently nonconducted atrial electrogram is virtually in the center of the diastolic interval between two QRS complexes. This immediately suggests a diagnosis of AV node reentry, in this case with 2:1 block below the level of the recorded His. This was indeed the case in this patient in whom slow pathway ablation eliminated tachycardia. Note, however, that this tracing in isolation does not rule out atrial tachycardia.

**Figure 3–16A**

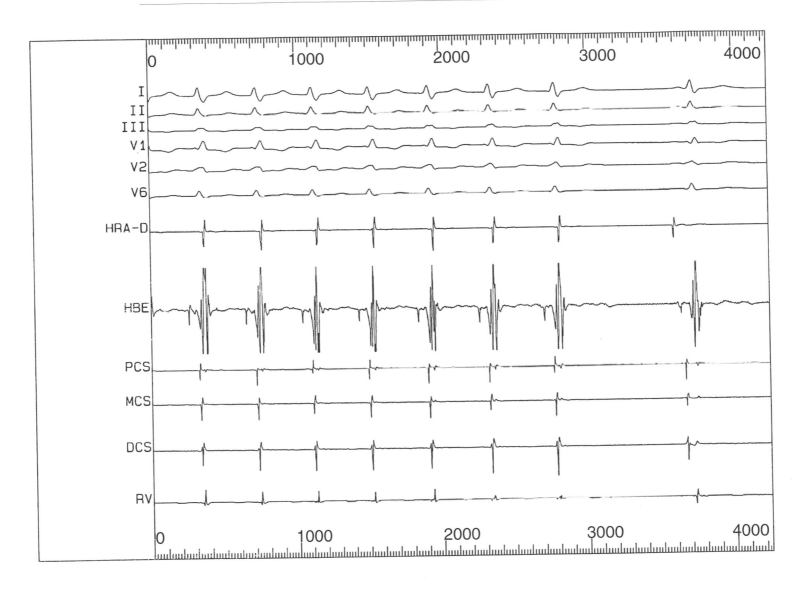

This is a 36-year-old woman with a history of palpitations. At EP study the observation shown here was made. What is the mechanism of tachycardia?

## *Figure 3–16B*

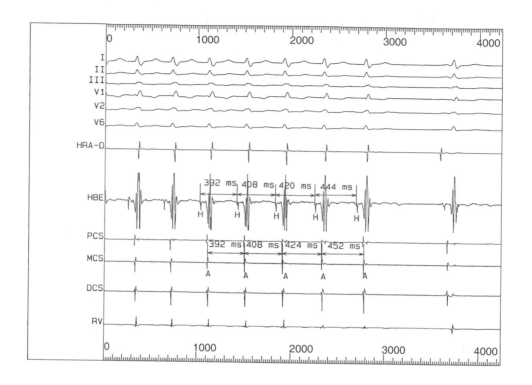

**Explanation:**

This patient has SVT with a relatively short VA interval. Of note, the activation sequence is low to high atrium. Thus, sinus tachycardia is excluded by the atrial activation sequence, and AV reentry is excluded by the short VA interval. AV nodal reentry and atrial tachycardia remain possibilities. This differential diagnosis often depends on demonstrating that the AV node is part of the tachycardia circuit, or that the atrium is not required. In this instance the AV node is implicated in the circuit. Note the progressive prolongation of tachycardia cycle length as measured by the H–H intervals on the His bundle lead. These precede and predict subsequent changes in atrial cycle length, and the tachycardia terminates with an atrial electrogram that does not conduct to the AV node. This observation implies that the AV node is part of the tachycardia circuit, and the diagnosis is AV node reentry. Changes in AV node conduction have no effect on the rate of atrial tachycardia. One would not expect atrial tachycardia to terminate because of loss of AV node conduction, although this could happen fortuitously. Consistent termination of tachycardia without AV node conduction implicates the AV node as part of the circuit.

# *Figure 3–17A*

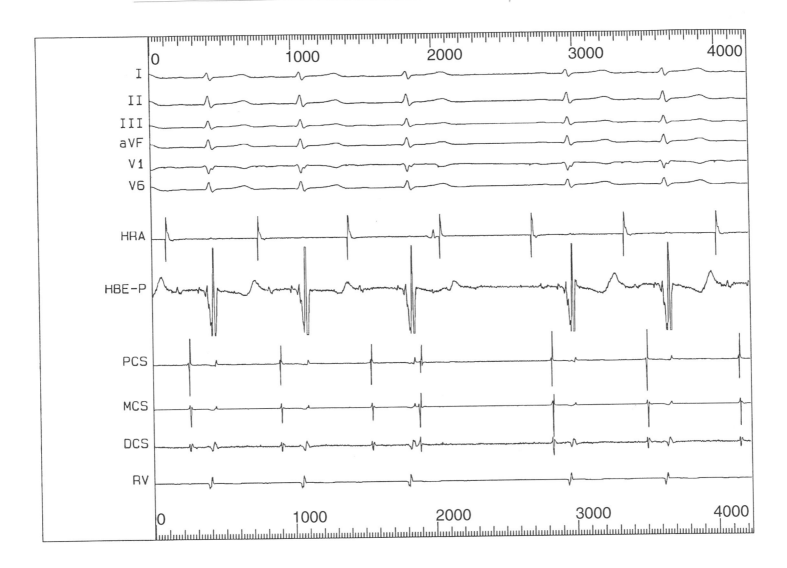

This patient has a history of documented paroxysmal SVT (PSVT). During atrial pacing the observation shown was noted. What is the likely mechanism of tachycardia? Why did the patient not have tachycardia? What would you do next to try to initiate tachycardia?

## Figure 3-17B

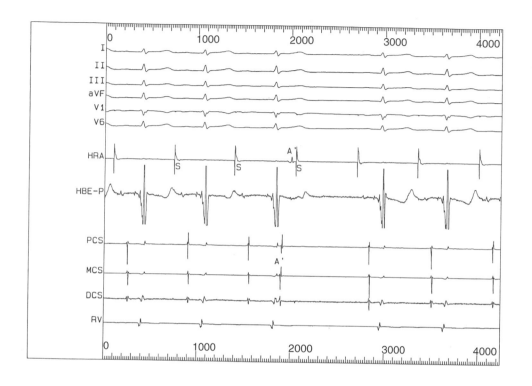

### Explanation:

During atrial pacing there is a progressive prolongation of the AH interval. After the third paced beat the drive train is interrupted by a premature atrial complex (A'). The activation sequence is eccentric, occurring first in the CS. Although this could be a premature atrial complex originating in the left atrium, the more likely diagnosis is an AV reentrant echo utilizing a concealed left-sided AP for retrograde conduction.

Tachycardia does not occur because the atrial echo does not conduct over the AV node. This is not surprising since there was progressive prolongation of the AH interval during pacing, sug-

gesting a Wenckebach sequence, and the AV reentrant echo has an even shorter interval than the drive complexes. Note that retrograde conduction over the AP occurred only after a substantial AV nodal delay on the third paced beat. It is not known whether there is complete anterograde block in the retrograde concealed AP or some degree of penetrance. Regardless, there must be a requisite delay before retrograde conduction can occur over the AP, and this is provided by the critically prolonged AH interval from the third paced beat. To initiate sustained tachycardia, isoproterenol was given and sustained AV reentry was initiated during atrial pacing (Fig. 3-17C).

## Figure 3–17C

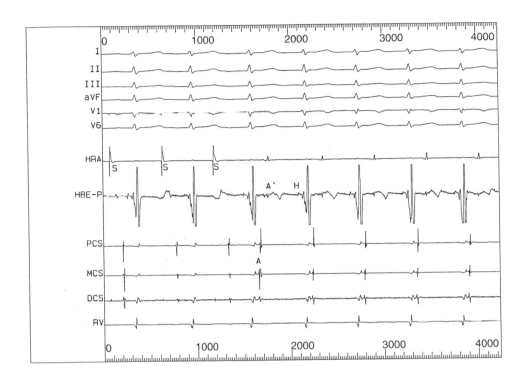

*Figure 3–18A*

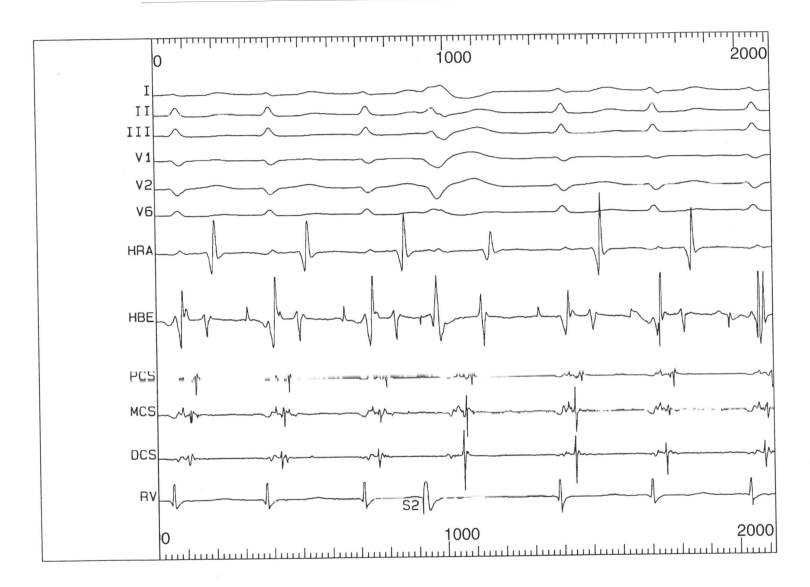

A premature ventricular complex was introduced during tachycardia.
Has the mechanism of tachycardia been identified?

3  NARROW QRS TACHYCARDIA

# Figure 3–18B

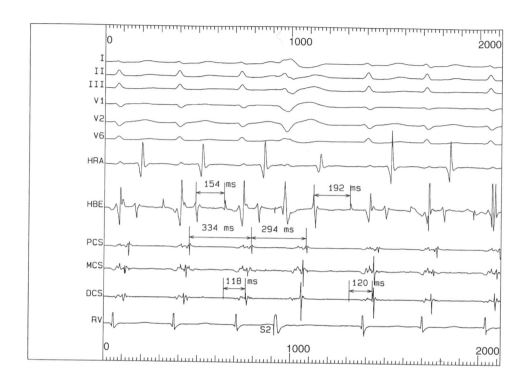

## Explanation:

The patient has a regular SVT with an eccentric atrial activation sequence with earliest activation occurring on the distal CS electrode positioned at the left lateral atrium. The differential diagnosis is a left atrial tachycardia versus AV reentry. The PVC preexcites the atrium during tachycardia, identifying the presence of a left-sided AP. Preexcitation of the atrium does not confirm participation of the pathway during tachycardia. This is true even though the activation sequence is similar for the tachycardia and preexcited atrial complexes. One could postulate the very unlikely occurrence of a left-sided atrial tachycardia originating in an area very near the left-sided

AP. Additional data in this figure essentially confirm the diagnosis of AV reentry. Note that the premature atrial complex (294 ms) following the premature ventricular complex causes a subsequent prolongation in AV nodal conduction time from 154 to 192 ms. Regardless, the His to local atrial interval is essentially unchanged from 118 to 120 ms. The "marriage" of the local atrial electrogram to the preceding His bundle deflection regardless of AV node conduction time would not be anticipated in an atrial tachycardia. Since fortuitous resetting of the atrial interval during an atrial tachycardia could produce the same result for a single premature complex, multiple intervals should be measured to confirm the diagnosis.

## Figure 3–19A

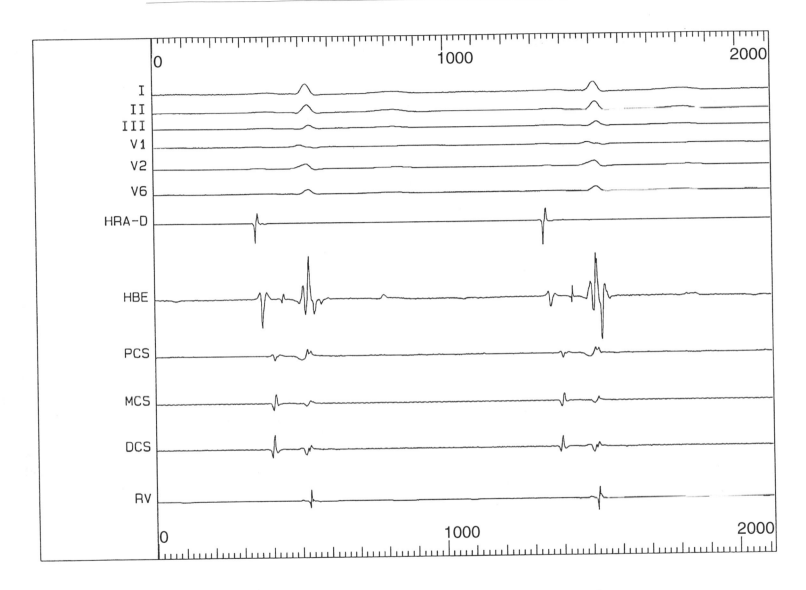

This patient has a history of palpitations and presyncope. Are there any clues to the diagnosis identified in this figure?

# Figure 3–19B

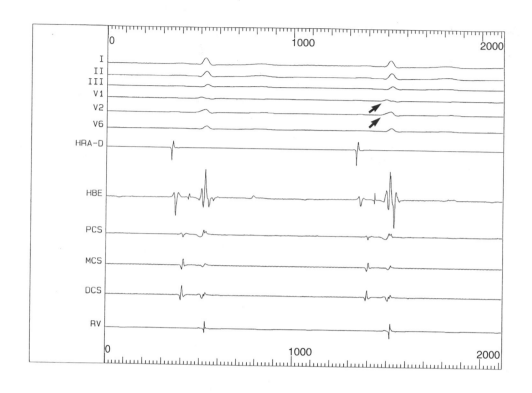

## Explanation:

Two subtle observations are suggestive of Wolff-Parkinson-White syndrome. First, the initial portion of the QRS complex in V1 and V2 (*arrows*) is abnormal and could represent preexcitation. Second, the HV interval is short, measuring 30 ms. The relatively short AH interval precluded more marked preexcitation during sinus rhythm in this patient. Note the rapid preexcited ventricular response during atrial fibrillation in Fig. 3–19C, which was associated with hypotension and dizziness, and likely was the cause of the patient's presyncopal episode.

**Figure 3–19C**

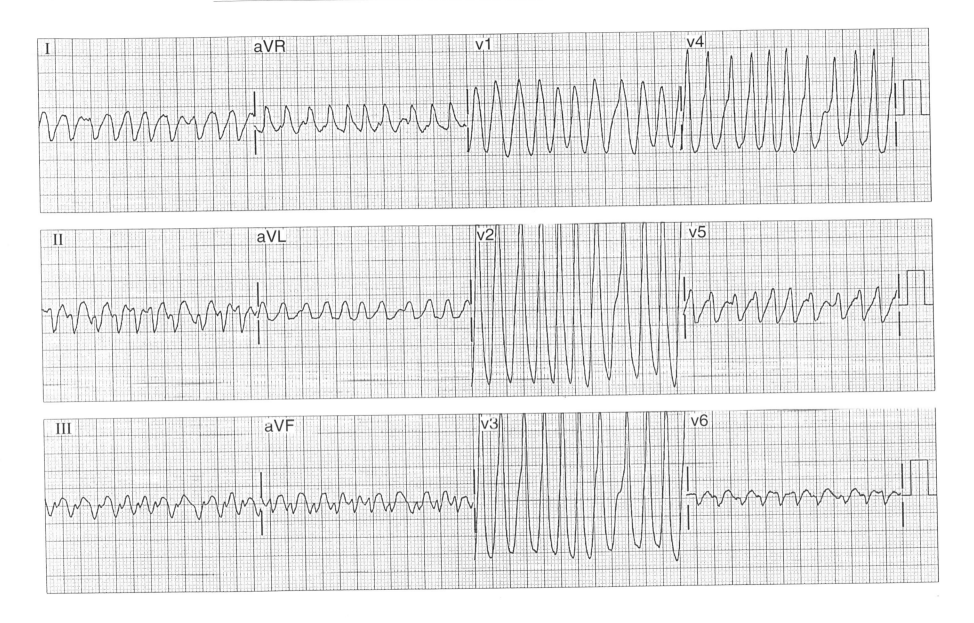

## Figure 3–20A

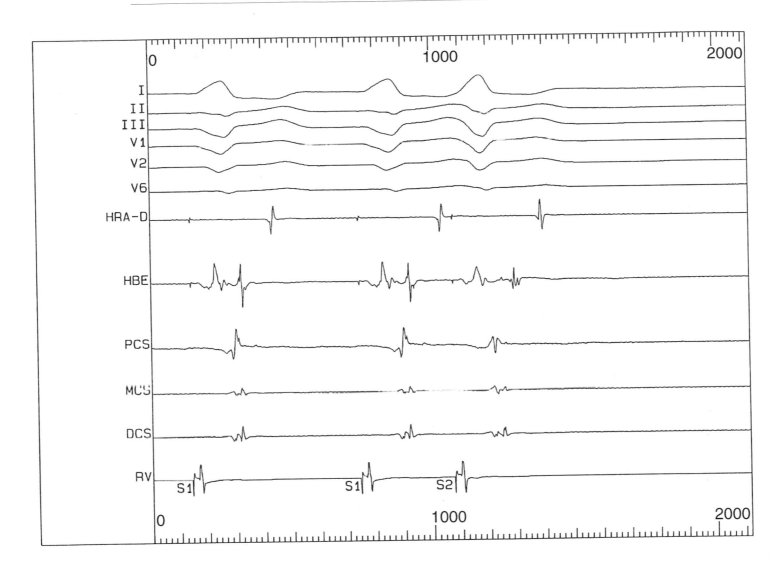

The tracing was recorded during premature ventricular stimulation in a patient with documented SVT. What is the likely mechanism of tachycardia? Why was it not initiated? What pacing maneuvers would help to initiate tachycardia?

## Figure 3–20B

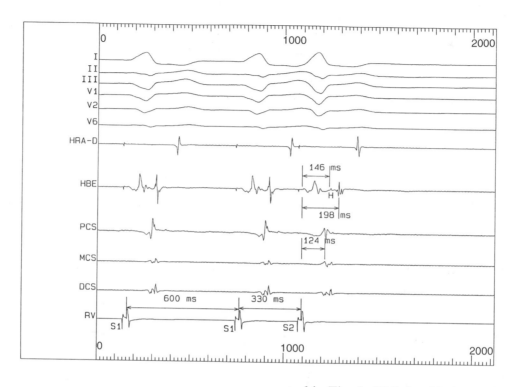

## Explanation:

The patient has a left free wall AP. This is confirmed during premature ventricular stimulation. Note that activation of the atrial electrogram in the proximal CS lead precedes activation of a retrograde His potential. The CS VA interval of 124 ms is substantially shorter than the 198-ms interval recorded in the His bundle electrogram. Tachycardia does not occur because the PVC conducted retrogradely into the AV node, which precluded subsequent anterograde AV nodal conduction.

Initiation of AV reentry during programmed ventricular stimulation requires minimal to no retrograde conduction into the AV node, that is, unidirectional block. The simplest method to achieve this goal is to introduce progressively shorter premature intervals as

noted in Fig. 3–20C. In this instance tachycardia is initiated with an S1S2 interval of 320 ms, and the VA conduction times on the CS and His bundle leads are similar to those in Fig. 3–20B. Note that a retrograde His deflection is not present, suggesting block in the HPS with this PVC. The similar VA conduction times on the His bundle electrogram with both PVCs strongly suggests that they were activated by conduction proceeding from the left atrium to the septum over the AP. Other methods to initiate AV reentry during ventricular pacing include multiple premature complexes, burst ventricular pacing, and pacing at slower cycle lengths. At slower paced cycle lengths, the refractoriness of the HPS often prolongs more than the AP, allowing block in the HPS to occur while conduction can still proceed over the AP.

# *Figure 3–20C*

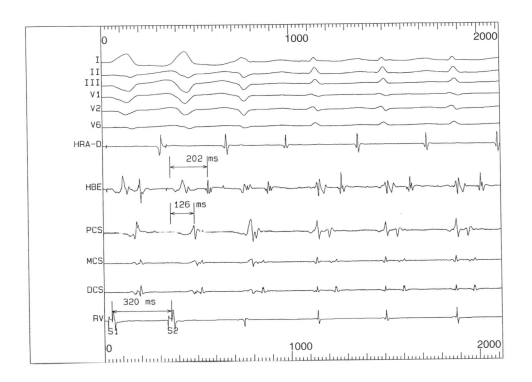

## *Figure 3–21A*

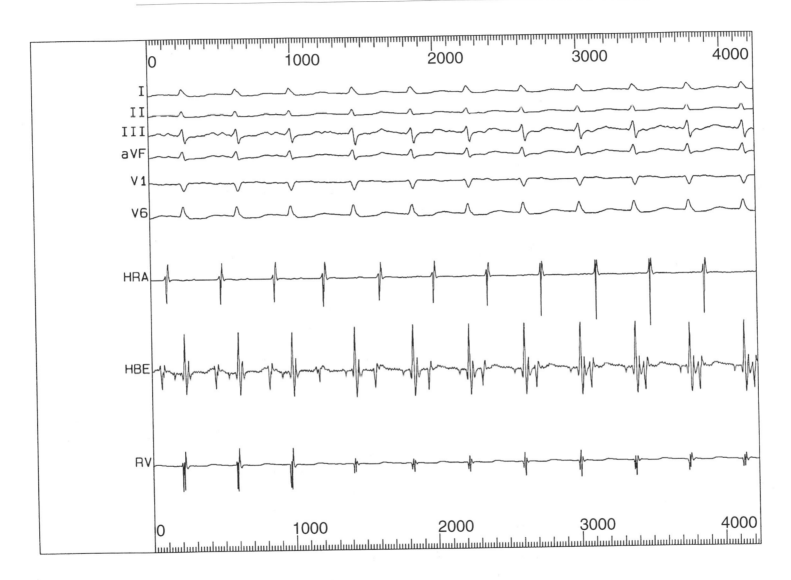

This patient had nearly incessant tachycardia. What is the likely mechanism?

# Figure 3–21B

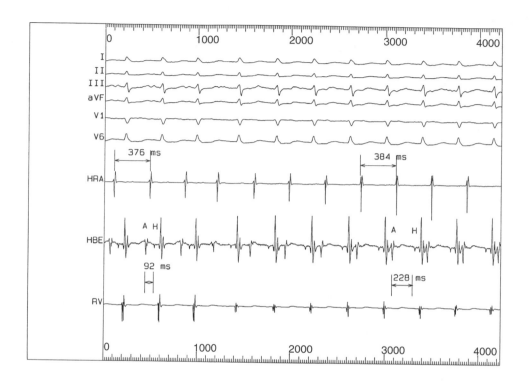

## Explanation:

This is a SVT with a low to high atrial activation pattern. There is minimal variability in the atrial cycle length. Differential diagnosis is AV node reentry, AV reentry, and atrial tachycardia. Note that the AH interval progressively lengthens from 92 to 228 ms in this tracing. With lengthening of the AH interval, there is a shortening of the measured VA interval. Yet, there is minimal change in the atrial cycle length. This is typical of atrial tachycardia and essentially excludes AV and AV node reentry. It is conceivable that one could have AV node reentry with the circuit totally proximal to the area of AV nodal conduction delay. If this occurred in the interatrial septum, especially along the tricuspid annulus, it would be impossible to differentiate from a septal tachycardia in this location. There have to be some rules established to differentiate these arrhythmias. In general, when marked changes in the AH interval occur without corresponding changes in atrial cycle length, we exclude the AV node as a significant part of the tachycardia circuit. Programmed stimulation techniques are also useful to support the diagnosis of atrial tachycardia. Initiation with PACs of tachycardia with a similar cycle length but with marked variability in AH interval, or without AV node conduction, suggests atrial tachycardia. Continuation of tachycardia without changes in atrial cycle length when PVCs are introduced and cause marked AH variation also supports the diagnosis of atrial tachycardia.

# Figure 3–22A

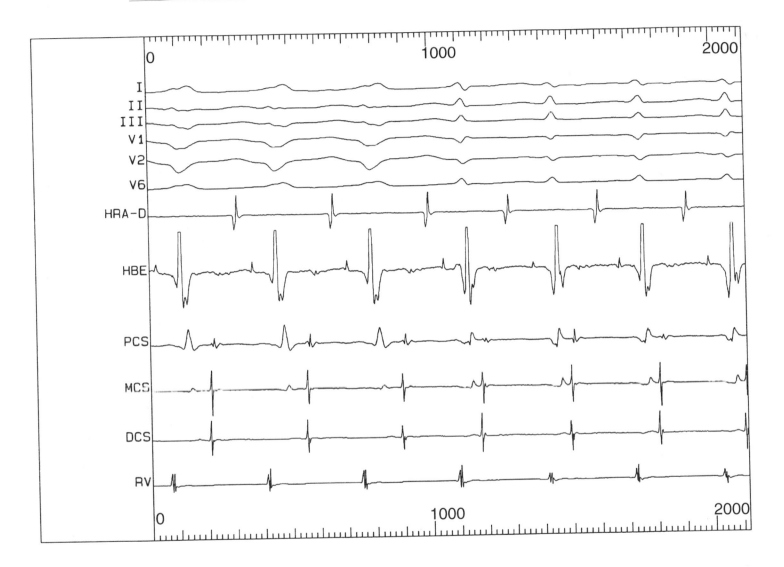

This tracing contains many interesting electrophysiologic observations. Are there one or two tachycardias present? Is there proof of the tachycardia mechanism? Why is there a change in atrial cycle length, and why isn't it larger?

# Figure 3-22B

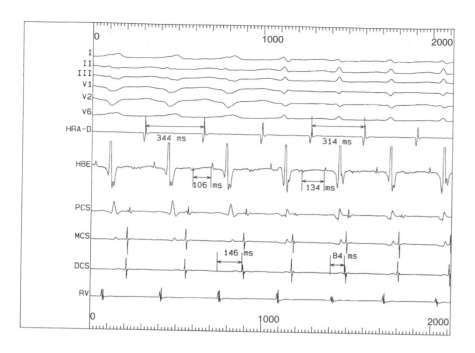

**Explanation:**

This patient has one tachycardia, AV reentry using a left-sided AP for retrograde conduction. During induction of tachycardia, the patient frequently had a short run of LBBB aberrancy that normalized. This probably represents progressive shortening of the refractory period of the left bundle branch to allow conduction to occur, rather than transseptal concealed conduction, which typically is long lasting. With normalization of the QRS, the VA interval shortens from 146 to 84 ms. This confirms participation of the left-sided AP in the tachycardia circuit. This sudden shortening of the VA interval also results in a shortened AA interval, followed by prolongation of the AH interval from 106 to 134 ms. Thus, although the atrial cycle length is shortened from 344 to 314 ms, the amount of cycle length decrease is mitigated by the concomitant increase in AH interval. In approximately 10 to 15% of patients, there is an increase in AH interval that approximates the shortening of VA interval and no change in tachycardia cycle length occurs. Thus, the change in VA interval is the critical measurement and not change in cycle length.

When analyzing electrocardiograms, one does not have the advantage of accurately measuring VA intervals in most cases. Thus, in this situation a difference in tachycardia cycle length between bundle branch block and narrow QRS complex morphology is the critical diagnostic point that implicates an AP as part of the tachycardia circuit. However, constant cycle length in this situation never excludes an AP as part of the tachycardia circuit. When a change in cycle length occurs it is typically stated that the AP is ipsilateral to the blocked bundle branch, yet there is an exception to this "rule." A patient could have marked prolongation of His-Purkinje conduction time with the bundle branch block complex, which shortens substantially with normalization of the QRS complex. In this situation the tachycardia cycle length might decrease because His-Purkinje conduction is part of the tachycardia cycle length. This would occur at any location of the AP. Regardless, this observation does implicate an AP in the tachycardia circuit.

## Figure 3–23A

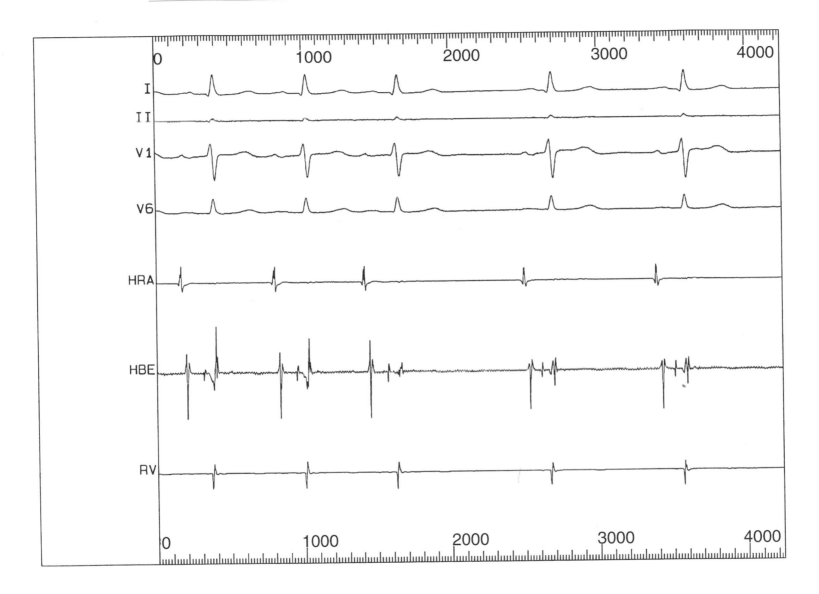

What is the likely mechanism of tachycardia on the left side of this figure?

## *Figure 3–23B*

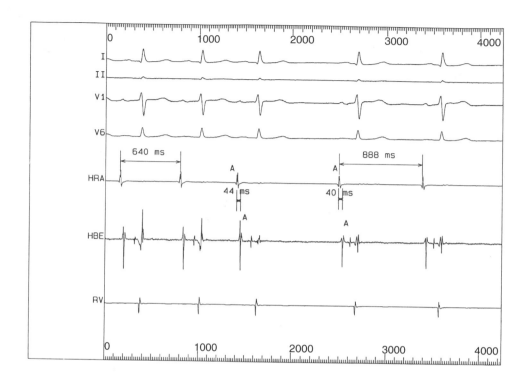

### Explanation:

This patient had a more rapid PSVT, but at EP study another form of tachycardia was also induced, and was never sustained. Note that the atrial activation sequence during tachycardia (cycle length of 640 ms) is nearly identical to that in sinus rhythm (cycle length of 888 ms). Although only two intracardiac leads are present, comparison of the P waves on the surface ECG shows that they are nearly identical. This likely represents sinus node reentry, although one can never exclude an atrial tachycardia originating within a few millimeters of the sinus node. Nonsustained sinus node reentry is commonly initiated at EP study. In general, it is not an arrhythmia requiring treatment.

## Figure 3–24A

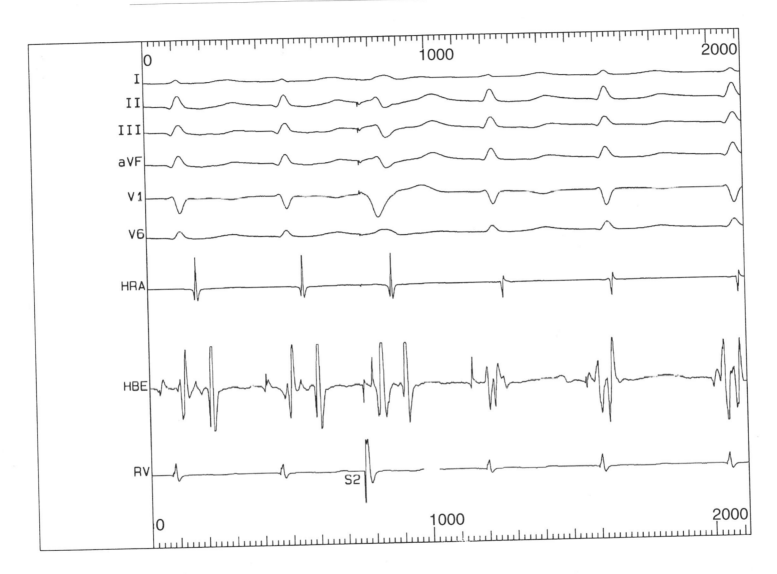

This observation occurred during SVT after introduction of a PVC.
Explain the finding.

*Figure 3–24B*

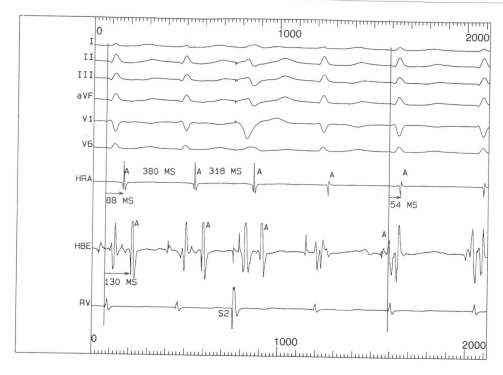

## Explanation:

The PVC is introduced prior to activation of the His bundle electrogram, and does not change the timing of the HH interval. The ventricle to high right atrium and His bundle atrium intervals are 88 and 130 ms, respectively. Prior to introduction of the PVC, there is no way to know whether the "VA" interval actually represents conduction from ventricle to atrium or if it is really AV conduction. In fact, there appears to be a high to low atrial activation sequence. One must remember that electrodes positioned in the high lateral right atrial area also record atrial activity from the lateral right atrium. Thus, if retrograde conduction occurs over a right lateral AP, activation on the high right atrial catheter can precede activation of the interatrial septum. This gives the illusion of a high to low atrial activation sequence.

The PVC clearly preexcites the atrium and shortens the cycle length from 380 to 318 ms without a change in the atrial activation sequence. Since the PVC was introduced at a time when the His bundle was refractory, the tachycardia mechanism most likely is AV reentry and the presumption is that a right lateral AP is present. Note that the QRS complex after the PVC is associated with a change in atrial activation sequence. The PVC "creates" a PAC (equivalent to atrial extrastimulus) and there is prolongation of the AH interval. The prolonged AH interval is followed by early atrial activation in the interatrial septum. The ventricle to high right atrium interval shortens to 54 ms, but is preceded by atrial septal activation. This patient now has AV node reentry with a slow anterograde and fast retrograde conduction pattern. Both arrhythmias were sustained and required ablation.

# *Figure 3–25A*

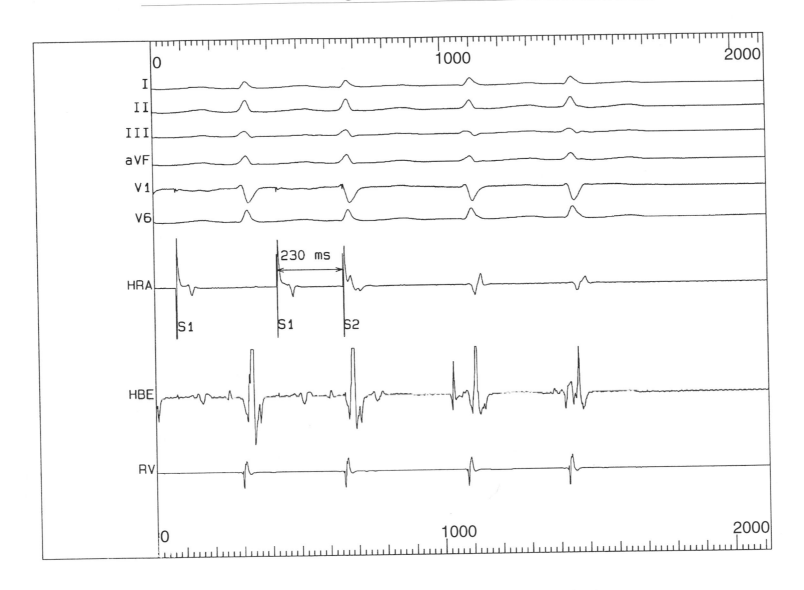

This patient has documented SVT. At EP study in the baseline state, the observation shown in the tracing was made. What is the likely mechanism of tachycardia?

# *Figure 3-25B*

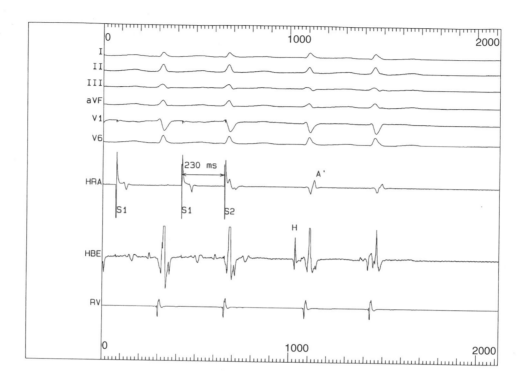

## Explanation:

A premature atrial complex of 230 ms conducts with a long AH interval and is followed by two subsequent atrial complexes. The VA interval is too short for AV reentry. Thus, the mechanism is either atrial tachycardia or AV node reentry. The echo complexes never terminated with conduction to the His bundle. This strongly suggests that the AV node is part of the tachycardia circuit, since termination of atrial tachycardia is not coupled to AV node conduc-tion. A useful technique is to try to establish a premature atrial coupling interval at which there is intermittent conduction to the His bundle. This is noted in Figs. 3-25B and 3-25C. The same coupling interval repeated many times produced atrial echoes only when His bundle activation occurred, strongly suggesting that AV nodal conduction was necessary for the atrial echo, implicating the AV node as part of the circuit. In the presence of isoproterenol, sustained AV node reentry was initiated.

# Figure 3–25C

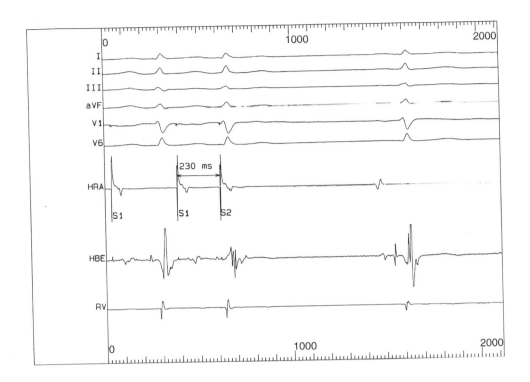

# Figure 3–26A

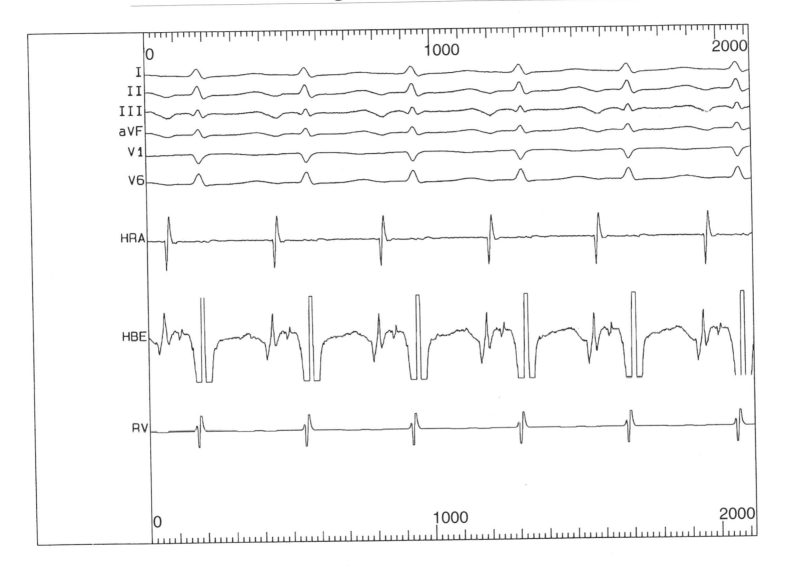

This record was taken during EP study of a patient with a long RP tachycardia. What is the differential diagnosis, and what techniques could you use to confirm the diagnosis without additional catheter placement?

*Figure 3–26B*

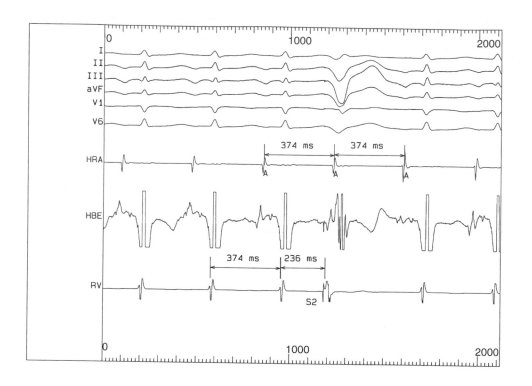

**Explanation:**

The differential diagnosis in a long RP tachycardia includes atrial tachycardia, AV reentry using an AP with slow retrograde conduction characteristics, and AV node reentry with slow retrograde and fast anterograde AV nodal conduction. Figure 3–26B demonstrates introduction of a very close-coupled PVC during tachycardia. No preexcitation occurs and the preexcitation index is greater than 138 ms, inconsistent with conduction over an AP. However, this does not absolutely rule out AV reentry. Lack of atrial preexcitation during programmed right ventricular stimulation near the coronary sinus os area makes a diagnosis of AV reentry even less likely. The likely differential is atrial tachycardia versus AV node reentry. Figure 3–26C shows termination of tachycardia with two closely coupled PVCs without any preceding change in the tachycardia cycle length, and without any conduction of the PVCs to the atrium. This was a reproducible finding and rules out atrial tachycardia. The resultant diagnosis is AV node reentry. CS catheterization was performed during this study and confirmed concentric retrograde atrial activation.

Figure 3–26C

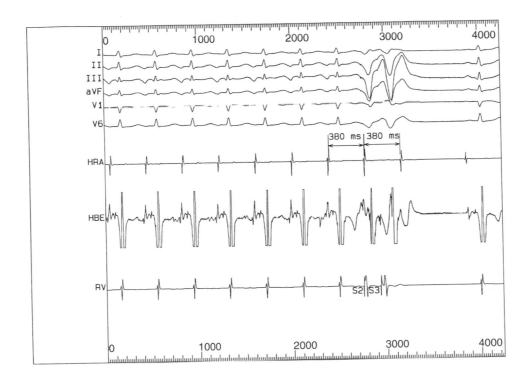

# Chapter 4

# *Wide QRS Complex Tachycardia*

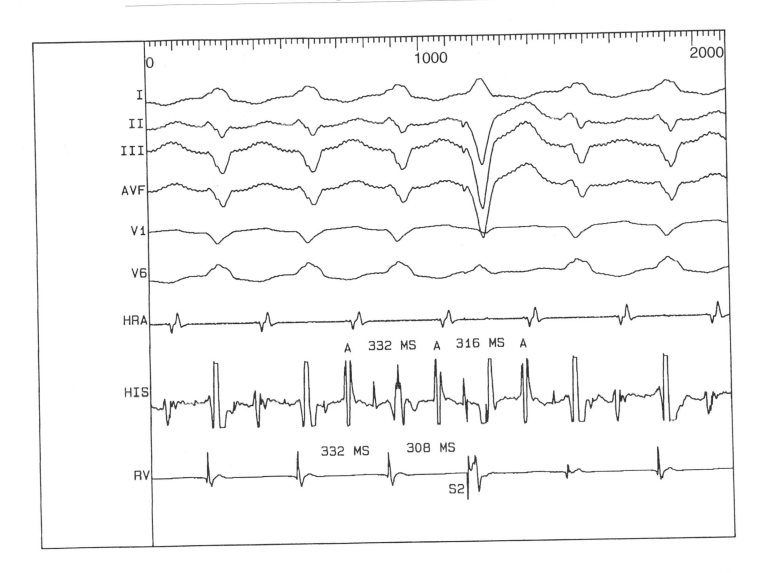

## Figure 4–1A

This 32-year-old man presented with a wide QRS complex tachycardia. At EP study the observation shown was made. What is the probable mechanism of tachycardia? What is the likely tachycardia circuit in this patient?

# Figure 4–1B

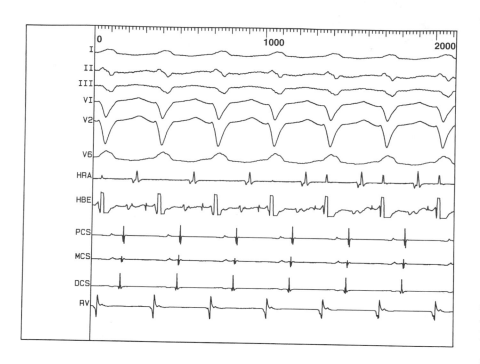

## Figure 4–1B

**Explanation:**

This figure demonstrates tachycardia with a CS lead in place, which was omitted in Fig. 4–1A. Note that there is eccentric atrial activation with earliest atrial activation at the distal CS electrode. The HV interval is normal. Thus, this is either a left atrial tachycardia or AV reentry utilizing a left-sided AP (Chapter 1, Table 1–7). Analysis of Fig. 4–1A demonstrates preexcitation of the atrium with a PVC introduced at a time when the His bundle is refractory. Thus, a left-sided AP is present and in this patient was involved in the tachycardia circuit. This observation alone does not absolutely exclude a coexisting atrial tachycardia.

The preexcitation index (PI) is a helpful adjunct to locate the site of the AP. It is determined by introducing progressively more premature right ventricular extrastimuli during tachycardia. The PI is calculated by subtracting the longest premature interval ($V_1 V_2$) that preexcites the atrium from the tachycardia cycle length ($V_1 V_1$). During a narrow QRS complex tachycardia, a relatively late-coupled $V_1V_2$ that preexcites the atrium (short PI) is typical for a right-sided or septal AP, and a PI <45 ms essentially excludes a left-sided AP. The PI of slow/fast AV node reentry is almost always > 90 ms.

In Fig. 4–1A, the preexcitation index is 24 ms (332 − 308 ms). Note that this patient has LBBB aberrancy. In this situation the ventricle is activated anterogradely over the right bundle branch, which exits near the moderator band in the right ventricular apex. The PVC has a morphology consistent with right ventricular apical pacing. Thus, the right ventricular catheter is near the tachycardia circuit, which now incorporates the right ventricular endocardium. During narrow QRS complex tachycardias, the premature ventricular complex conducts transseptally to enter the tachycardia circuit in a patient with a left-sided AP, and the PI is much longer.

In summary, a diagnosis of AV reentry was reasonable from Fig. 4–1A, but the location of the AP could not be determined from just this figure.

# *Figure 4–2A*

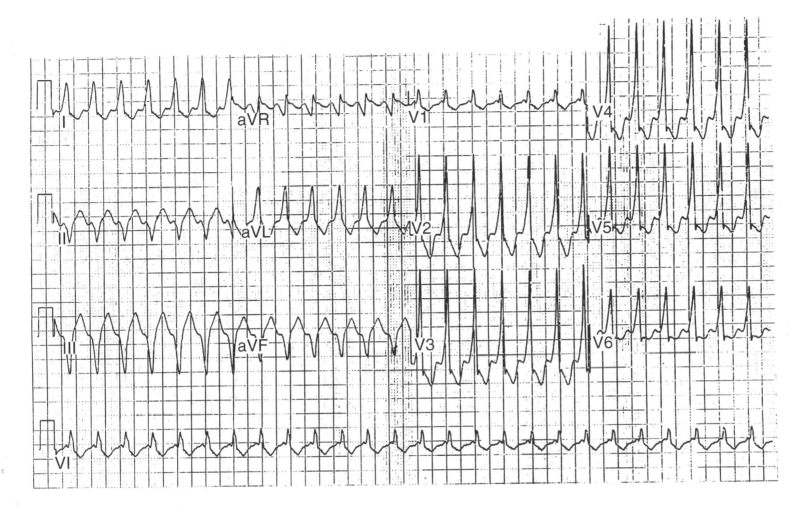

A 45-year-old man presents to the emergency room with a history of 2 hours of palpitations. A 12-lead electrocardiogram was recorded and is shown in Fig. 4–2A. What is the differential diagnosis? While taking the patient's history, what is probably the most important question you can ask to differentiate the mechanism of tachycardia? Does hemodynamic stability in this patient help to differentiate supraventricular from ventricular tachycardia?

4  WIDE QRS COMPLEX TACHYCARDIA

# Figure 4–2B

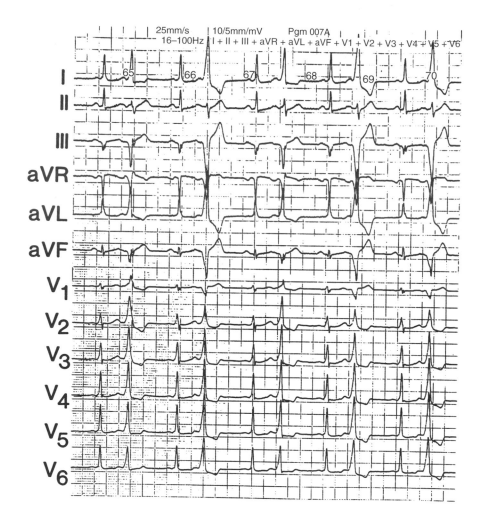

25mm/s 10/5mm/mV Pgm 007A
16–100Hz I + II + III + aVR + aVL + aVF + V1 + V2 + V3 + V4 + V5 + V6

cal," and less likely to represent aberrancy. The presumptive diagnosis should be VT until proven otherwise. After tachycardia was terminated a simultaneous 12-lead ECG rhythm strip was obtained (Fig. 4–2B). Note that this patient has intermittent wide QRS complexes during sinus rhythm, but more than one wide QRS morphology is present. Complexes 2 and 6 are nearly identical to the QRS complexes noted in Fig. 4–2A. This strongly suggests that a preexcited tachycardia was present in Fig. 4–2A since the PR intervals of the wide complexes are constant. An alternative diagnosis that must be excluded is coupled PVCs giving the illusion of a constant PR interval. The presence of an AP can be confirmed at EP study. The preexcited QRS morphology suggests a left posterior AP location. In contrast, QRS complexes 4, 8, and 10 demonstrate a different wide QRS morphology, and the PR intervals are constant. This likely represents a second preexcited QRS morphology, and the 12-lead ECG is consistent with a posteroseptal AP position. In patients with more than one AP, a common combination is posteroseptal and left free wall. Ventricular tachycardia is always part of the differential diagnosis.

The most important question you can ask a patient with a wide QRS complex tachycardia is whether they have a history of heart disease. In this case the patient had no heart disease and this makes ventricular tachycardia a less likely possibility. Further, if the patient has had a history of sustained tachycardia since childhood, the diagnosis of Wolff-Parkinson-White (WPW) syndrome is even greater. The morphology "rules" to differentiate supraventricular from ventricular tachycardia in the presence of RBBB do not apply in the presence of preexcitation. Even though the QRS morphology is more suggestive of ventricular tachycardia in Fig. 4–2A, this is not helpful since a preexcited tachycardia is present.

Hemodynamic stability does not differentiate SVT from ventricular tachycardia.

## Explanation:

Figure 4–2A is a RBBB tachycardia without evidence of VA dissociation. The differential diagnosis is VT, SVT with aberrancy, and a preexcited tachycardia (Chapter 1, Table 1–4). The RBBB is "atypi-

*Figure 4–3A*

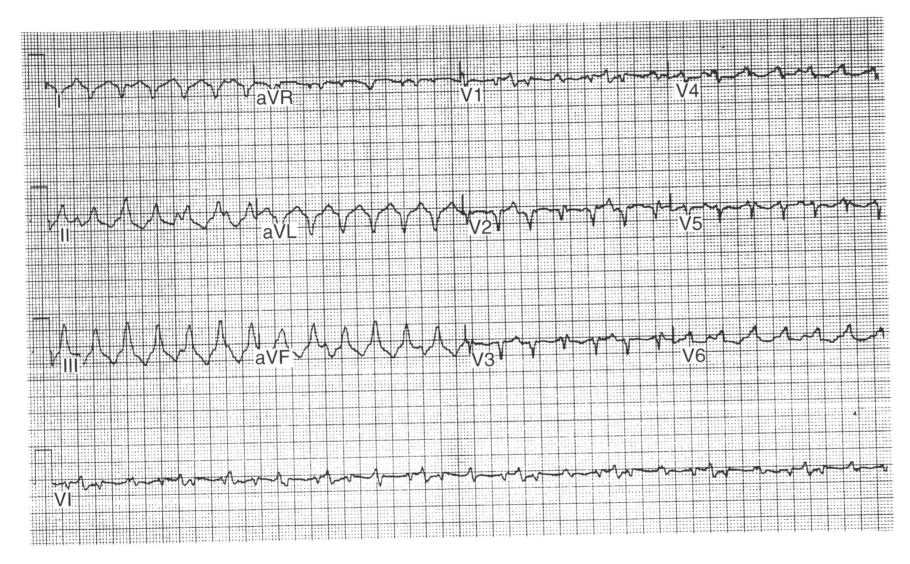

You are called to the emergency room to evaluate a patient who presents with palpitations. The 12-lead electrocardiogram in Fig. 4–3A was recorded during the patient's symptoms. What is the diagnosis?

## *Figure 4–3B*

**Sinus Rhythm**

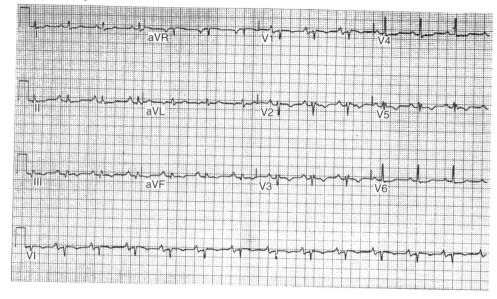

**Explanation:**

Analysis of the rhythm strip in $V_1$ of Fig. 4–3A demonstrates clear VA dissociation during tachycardia. The somewhat confusing pattern occurs because the P waves are actually larger in amplitude than the QRS complexes in this lead, as noted during sinus rhythm (Fig. 4–3B). This patient has ventricular tachycardia. The diagnosis might have been more difficult if only a rhythm strip of $V_1$ was available. Further, the QRS width in $V_1$ is barely 120 ms. This stresses the importance of obtaining a 12-lead electrocardiogram during tachycardia, and reserving judgment until multiple leads are analyzed.

## *Figure 4–4A*

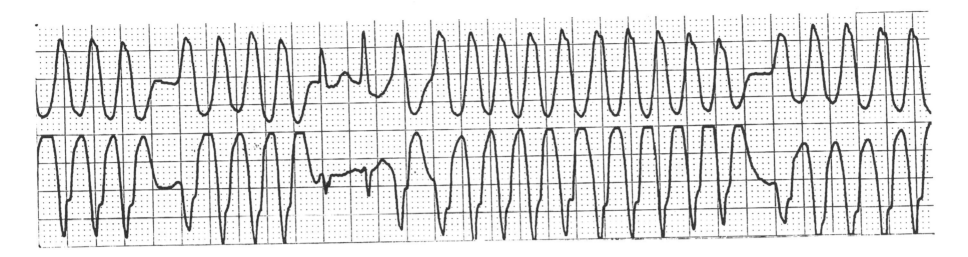

This patient was admitted with a history of syncope. During in-hospital monitoring, the rhythm shown was recorded during which the patient was hypotensive. What is the diagnosis?

# *Figure 4–4B*

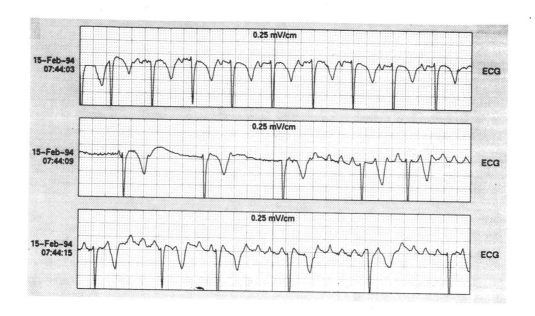

## Explanation:

A grossly irregular, rapid wide QRS complex tachycardia is nearly always atrial fibrillation with conduction over an AP. This patient had a posteroseptal AP that was successfully ablated at EP study. In Fig. 4–4*A*, there is a preexcited tachycardia with only two normally conducted QRS complexes. Degeneration of AV reentry to atrial fibrillation is the usual mechanism for AF in patients with WPW, and successful ablation of the AP prevents recurrences of AF in more than 90% of these patients. Clearly this was not the case in this patient as noted in Fig. 4–4*B*. The top rhythm strip reveals sinus rhythm and atrial flutter/fibrillation occurred spontaneously (middle rhythm strip). In patients in whom atrial fibrillation can be demonstrated as a primary arrhythmia, ablation of the AP should not be performed to prevent AF. However, prevention of conduction over the AP after ablation removes a potentially life-threatening situation in patients with rapid preexcited ventricular rates. If a patient demonstrated relatively poor conduction over the AP during atrial fibrillation, and antiarrhythmic drugs were selected to maintain sinus rhythm, ablation of the AP would offer little benefit to the patient.

## Figure 4–5A

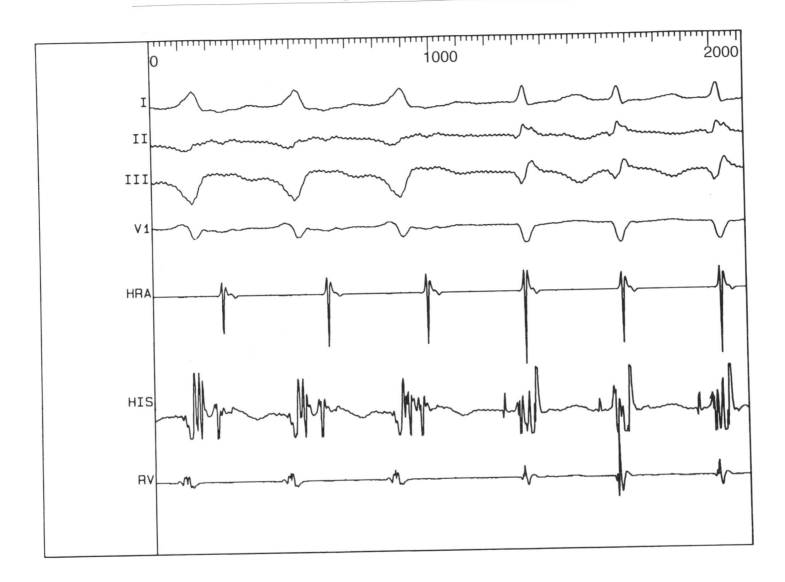

This middle-age man has a history of myocardial infarction. What is the diagnosis?

# *Figure 4–5B*

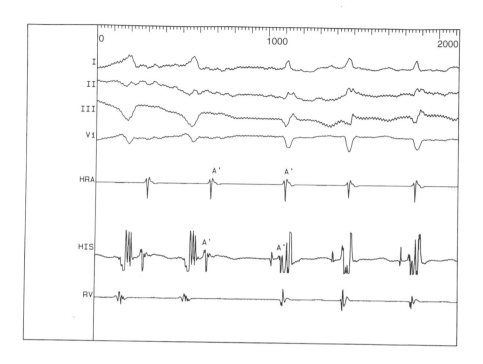

**Explanation:**

This figure demonstrates a wide QRS tachycardia followed by a narrow QRS tachycardia. There is no His deflection preceding ventricular activation in the wide QRS complexes, and the differential diagnosis is VT versus a preexcited tachycardia. This patient did not have ventricular preexcitation; thus, this is ventricular tachycardia with 1:1 VA conduction. Tachycardia spontaneously terminates and a narrow QRS complex tachycardia is induced (tachycardia-induced tachycardia) (Chapter 1, Table 1–3). There is a long AH interval followed by a change in retrograde atrial activation sequence. Atrial septal activation precedes high right atrial activation, and the His bundle atrial electrogram is located between the His bundle and QRS deflections. The VA interval is too short for AV reentry, and the most likely diagnosis is AV node reentry. At EP study both types of tachycardia could be independently induced. In addition, during continuous ECG inhospital monitoring, the patient had spontaneous episodes of tachycardia that demonstrated both a wide and narrow QRS complex morphology. The rate of the two tachycardias were very similar, causing confusion as to the appropriate diagnosis. These patients should undergo EP testing to confirm the diagnosis.

The importance of tachycardia-induced tachycardia cannot be overemphasized. Two particular situations need to be considered. First, it may explain a discrepancy in the clinical presentation. For example, patients may have documented, stable SVT but a history of syncope prior to recording the ECG. If ventricular tachycardia initiated SVT in these individuals, it is possible that syncope may have resulted from the ventricular tachycardia. Of course, patients may also have syncope with SVT. In someone with a history of heart disease this mechanism must be sought at EP testing. Second, in some individuals one arrhythmia always initiates the other arrhythmia. The most common example is AV reentry producing atrial fibrillation. Elimination of AV reentry can prevent both arrhythmias in this situation, and one does not need to treat the tachycardias as separate entities.

*Figure 4–6A*

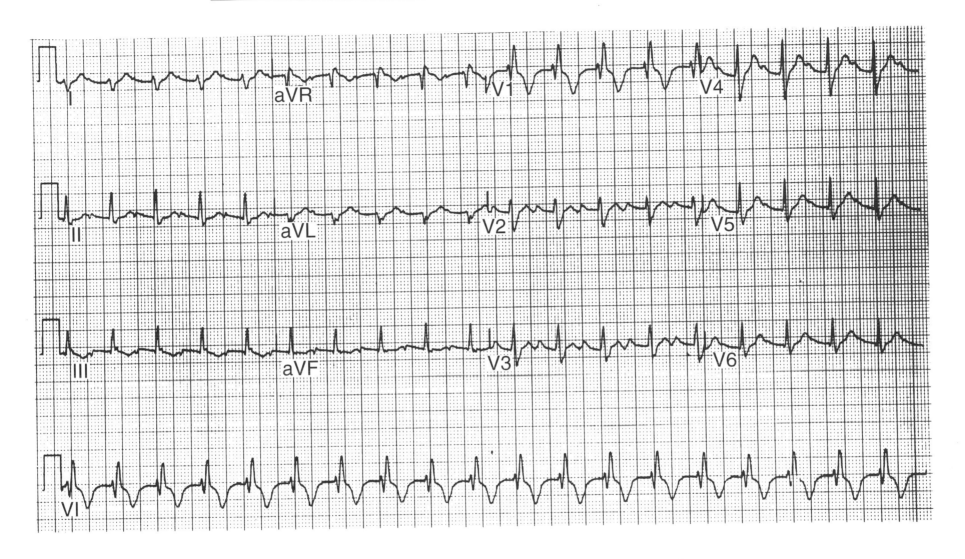

This patient has a history of palpitations and presyncope. What is the diagnosis?

# Figure 4–6B

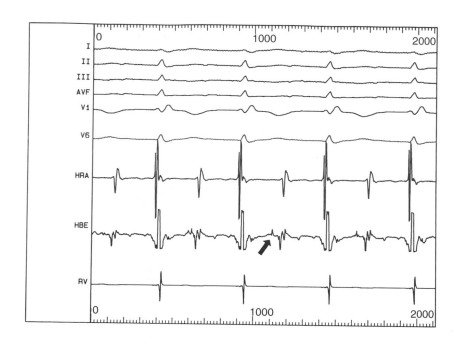

## Explanation:

In Fig. 4–6A, there is a typical triphasic RBBB tachycardia with atrial activity positioned almost exactly between the two QRS complexes. The QRS pattern suggests a supraventricular mechanism. ECG leads II, III, and aVF demonstrate P-wave activity equidistant between the two QRS complexes. In addition, the P waves suggest caudal-cranial activation and they are narrow. This is typical for atrial activation that originates in the interatrial septum. Thus, analysis of the 12-lead ECG in Fig. 4–6A reveals clues to diagnose AV node reentry with 2:1 block (Chapter 1, Table 1–6). However, EP study (Fig. 4–6B) was necessary for confirmation. The His bundle electrogram reveals 2:1 block below the His bundle deflection (*arrow*). There is a low to high atrial activation sequence, with early septal activation. This is typical for AV node reentry with 2:1 block below the His bundle.

# Figure 4–7A

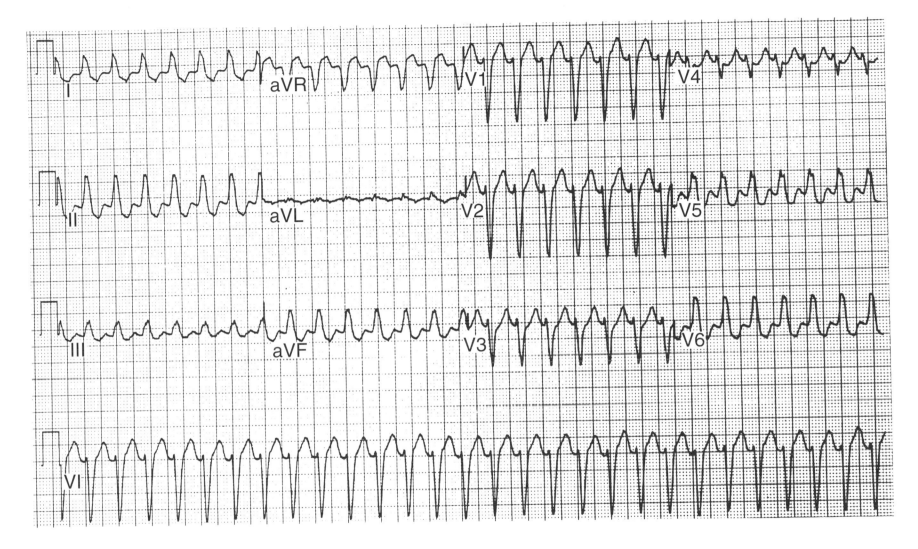

A 26-year-old man presents with a several-year history of intermittent palpitations. There is no history of heart disease. What is the differential diagnosis? Is this ventricular or supraventricular tachycardia?

# Figure 4–7B

**Figure 4–7B**

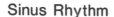

Sinus Rhythm

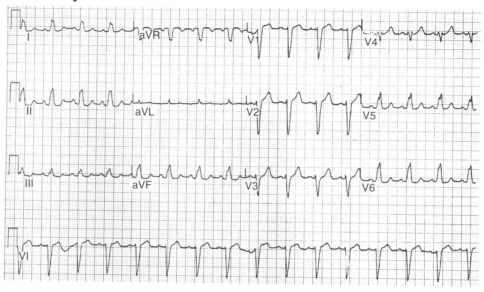

## Explanation:

Differentiation of LBBB tachycardias begins with careful analysis of the LBBB pattern. Activation of the ventricle over the right bundle yields a "typical" LBBB pattern as noted in this patient during sinus rhythm (Fig. 4–7B). The initial r wave in ECG leads $V_1$ and $V_2$ is narrow and followed by a rapidly conducted S wave. No Q wave is present in $V_6$. "Atypical" LBBB patterns can occur with activation of the right ventricle preceding the left ventricle and are quite variable. Examples are ventricular tachycardia as well as right-sided APs. If a typical LBBB pattern is present, the usual differential is any SVT with LBBB aberrancy, or unusual varieties of preexcited tachycardia such as atriofascicular and nodofascicular reentry. One exception might be bundle branch block reentry, but these patients typically have large dilated hearts and the QRS duration during tachycardia is often substantially prolonged (>160 ms).

Analysis of Fig. 4–7A reveals a typical LBBB pattern suggesting some form of supraventricular arrhythmia in this patient without a history of heart disease. Note the P-wave activity seen at the apex of the T wave in multiple leads, especially I, II, aVL, and aVF. The negative P wave in leads I and aVL suggests initiation of excitation in the left atrium. The differential diagnosis is a left atrial tachycardia with relatively long AV conduction time versus AV reentry using a concealed left-sided AP. The relatively long RP interval in this situation occurs because of the LBBB, which adds conduction time to the circuit since the right ventricle is activated prior to the left ventricle. Therefore, the P wave appears later than expected after the QRS complex.

At electrophysiologic study the tracing of Fig. 4–7C was obtained. Atrial activation is eccentric with earliest activity on the distal coronary sinus electrode. Pacing maneuvers confirmed a concealed left lateral AP and the patient had AV rentry.

*Figure 4-7C*

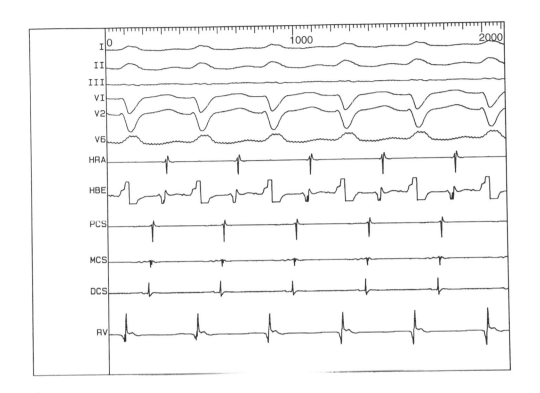

## *Figure 4–8A*

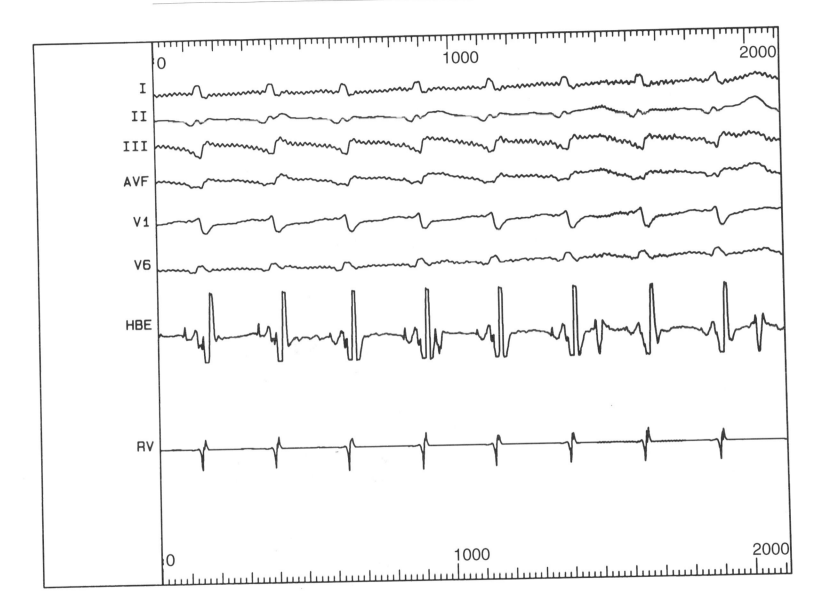

The rhythm shown was recorded at EP study. What is the diagnosis?

*Figure 4–8B*

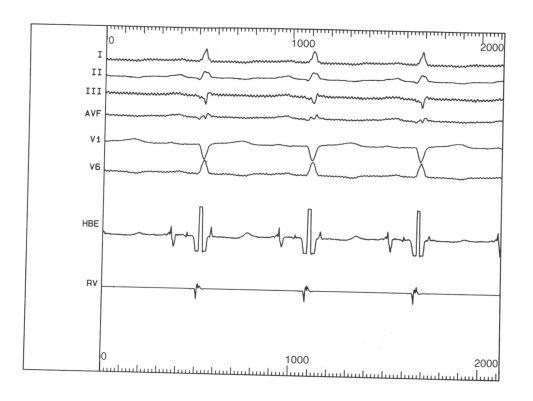

**Explanation:**

Figure 4–8*A* shows a regular tachycardia with the QRS duration slightly prolonged. A His bundle deflection is recorded before each ventricular activation on the His bundle lead. However, careful analysis reveals that the HV interval is actually short, with His activation occurring nearly simultaneously with the onset of ventricular activation as measured from the surface ECG (Chapter 1, Table 1–8). In addition, there is ventriculoatrial dissociation present, which is clearly demonstrated on the His bundle electrogram with the sixth and eighth QRS complex. The HV interval during sinus rhythm is noted in Fig. 4–8*B*, considerably longer than that recorded during tachycardia. Thus, the mere presence of a His bundle deflection preceding each QRS complex during tachycardia is not diagnostic of a supraventricular arrhythmia. The HV interval must be equal to or greater than the HV recorded without tachycardia, or the patient has a preexcited tachycardia or ventricular tachycardia. This patient had ventricular tachycardia with retrograde activation of the His bundle.

## Figure 4–9A

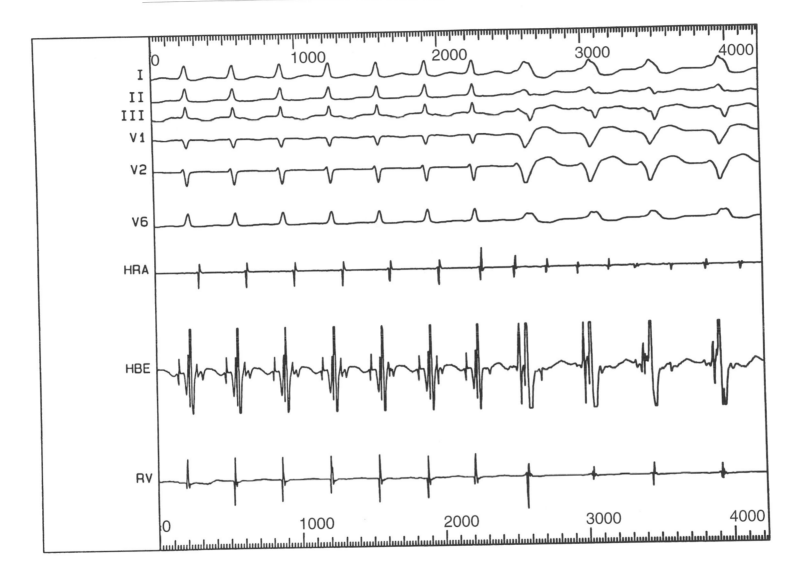

The tracing shown was observed at EP study in a young man without evidence of heart disease. What is the likely mechanism of tachycardia for both the narrow and wide QRS complex arrhythmias?

# *Figure 4–9B*

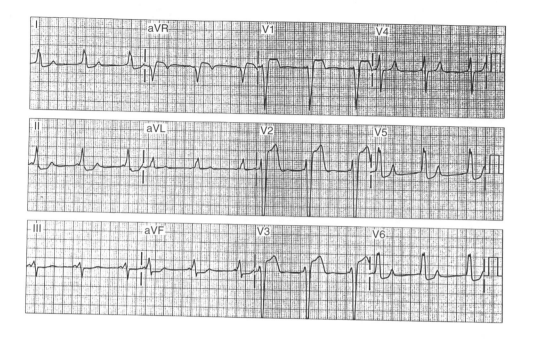

**Explanation:**

During sinus rhythm this patient exhibited ventricular preexcitation, and the location of the AP is near the right lateral AV groove (Fig. 4–9B). The tracing in Fig. 4–9A reveals a regular narrow QRS complex tachycardia that turns into an irregular wide QRS complex tachycardia. The narrow QRS tachycardia could be due to several mechanisms, including atrial tachycardia, AV node reentry, and AV reentry. The VA interval is longer than usual for AV node reentry, but certainly does not exclude this diagnosis. The male gender and younger age of the patient is more consistent with AV reentry.

Regardless, one cannot make a definitive statement regarding mechanism of tachycardia from this tracing alone.

The regular SVT degenerates into atrial fibrillation as noted by the high right atrial recording. Atrial fibrillation is associated with a wide QRS complex morphology, consistent with a right-sided AP. Further, a distinct His bundle deflection no longer precedes each ventricular depolarization during the wide QRS complex arrhythmia. Thus, this represents either a preexcited tachycardia or ventricular tachycardia, and not aberrancy. When one considers all the data, the most likely single diagnosis is AV reentry that degenerates into atrial fibrillation, producing a preexcited tachycardia.

# Figure 4–10A

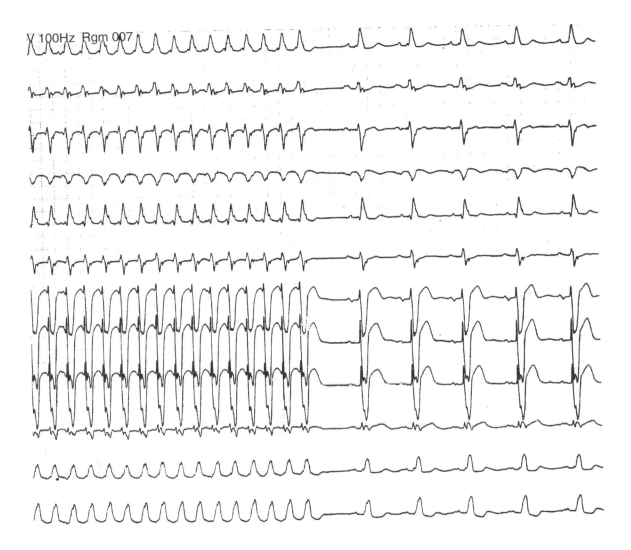

Y 100Hz Rgm 007

This patient with cardiomyopathy presents to the emergency room with hypotension and a history of syncope. A simultaneous 12-lead electrocardiogram is taken and the leads from top to bottom are I, II, III, aVR, aVL, aVF, and $V_1$ to $V_6$. The tachydardia spontaneously terminated. What is the differential diagnosis?

# *Figure 4–10B*

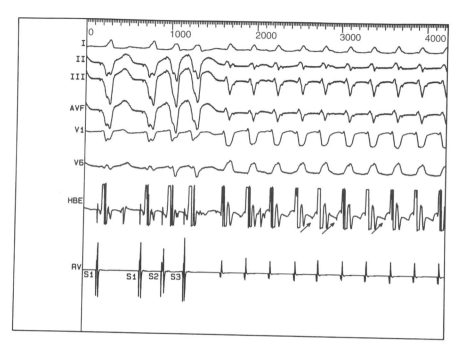

of a fast paced rate followed by a pause and then introduction of one or more extrastimuli. This theoretically produces divergence in refractoriness in the HPS and ventricle, allowing for retrograde block in the right bundle branch, transseptal conduction to the left bundle branch, and then reexcitation of the right bundle branch for initiation of tachycardia. Each QRS complex is preceded by a His potential with an HV interval typically equal to or greater than the HV measured in sinus rhythm. VA dissociation is the rule. In fact, this arrhythmia often occurs in patients with atrial fibrillation. Importantly, since the ventricle is activated over the right bundle branch, a "typical" LBBB morphology may be seen. This is well illustrated in Fig. 4–10*A* in which the patient has an underlying LBBB pattern that is nearly identical to that occurring during tachycardia on the left-hand portion of the figure.

Bundle branch reentry occurs almost exclusively in patients with dilated cardiomyopathies, ischemic or nonischemic, and the QRS duration during tachycardia is often >160 ms. Although ablation of the right bundle branch may prevent tachycardia in some of these patients, these individuals also have poor left ventricular function and may have other sustained ventricular arrhythmias. This should be evaluated very carefully before accepting right bundle branch ablation as a sole therapy for a particular patient.

## Explanation:

Careful analysis of lead I in Fig. 4–10*A* shows VA dissociation, a subtle finding in this tracing. There is an LBBB pattern during tachycardia that is nearly identical to that seen in sinus rhythm. These observations suggest bundle branch reentrant VT.

Figure 4–10*B* was obtained during EP testing in this patient. During ventricular drive, a second PVC initiated sustained VT with an identical ECG morphology as recorded in Fig. 4–10*A*. Note that there is VA dissociation. More important, His bundle deflections (*arrows*) occur prior to each QRS complex. The HV interval was slightly longer than that recorded during sinus rhythm. This patient had bundle branch reentrant VT. The typical EP findings are inducibility at EP study, sometimes requiring the unusual pacing protocol

# Figure 4–11A

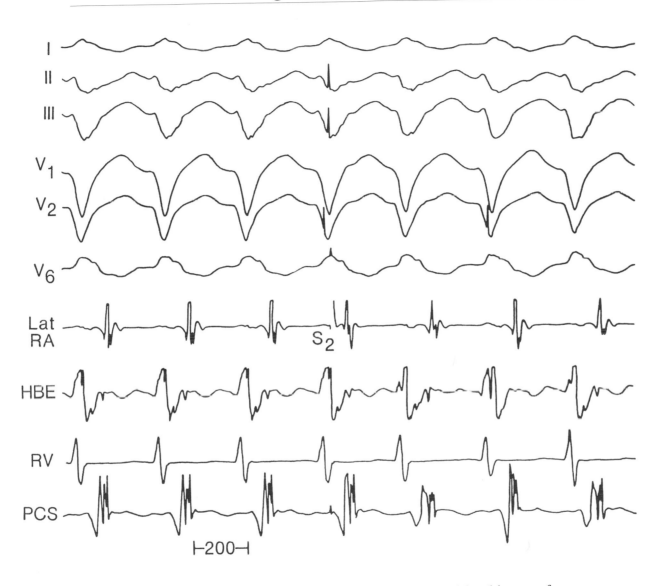

I

II

III

V₁

V₂

V₆

Lat RA

S₂

HBE

RV

PCS

⊢200⊣

This tracing was obtained at EP study in a patient with a history of wide QRS complex tachycardia. The proximal CS recording electrode was positioned at the os of the CS. What is the diagnosis?

# Figure 4-11B

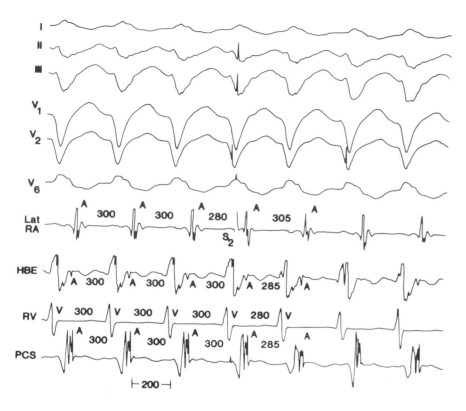

VT versus preexcited tachycardia. The QRS morphology demonstrates an atypical LBBB pattern that is consistent with either diagnosis. The tachycardia cycle length is 300 ms, and a 20-ms premature atrial stimulus is introduced in the lateral right atrium. This premature complex does not affect septal activation as noted by a lack of change in the AA interval on the His bundle electrogram. However, the PAC shortens the VV interval, with an identical QRS morphology. This confirms AV activation over an AP during tachycardia. Although VT has been eliminated, the mechanism of tachycardia requires further analysis of this tracing.

The preexcited tachycardia could be antidromic reentry utilizing a right free wall AP for anterograde conduction and the normal VA conduction system for retrograde activation, AP–AP tachycardia using a septal AP for retrograde conduction, bystander AP conduction during arrhythmias such as AV node reentry, and septal atrial tachycardia, or nodoventricular reentry. Careful measurement of the His bundle AA interval following shortening of the VV interval shows a decrease from 300 to 285 ms. Atrial preexcitation of the ventricle without affecting the septal atrial sequence eliminates nodoventricular reentry. Likewise, "reset" of a septal atrial tachycardia would not occur since the initial atrial activation sequence was unperturbed by the PAC. AV node reentry with bystander participation is also excluded. The preexcited ventricular response of only 20 ms (280 ms) produces a shortening of the subsequent septal AA interval. Although preexcitation of the atrium during AV node reentry can occur, the PI is >90 ms. In this case the PI would be only 20 ms, too short for AV node reentry. The final differential diagnosis is true antidromic tachycardia utilizing the normal VA conduction system for retrograde activation versus retrograde conduction over a second AP located in the septum. This patient had antidromic tachycardia, the most common diagnosis with this presentation.

## Explanation:

A regular wide QRS complex tachycardia is present with 1:1 VA association. Atrial activation sequence demonstrates earliest activity in the interatrial septum, as recorded on the His bundle lead. There is no obvious His bundle deflection preceding each QRS complex, and the His bundle electrode was recording a good His potential prior to initiation of tachycardia. Thus, the differential diagnosis is

## Figure 4–12A

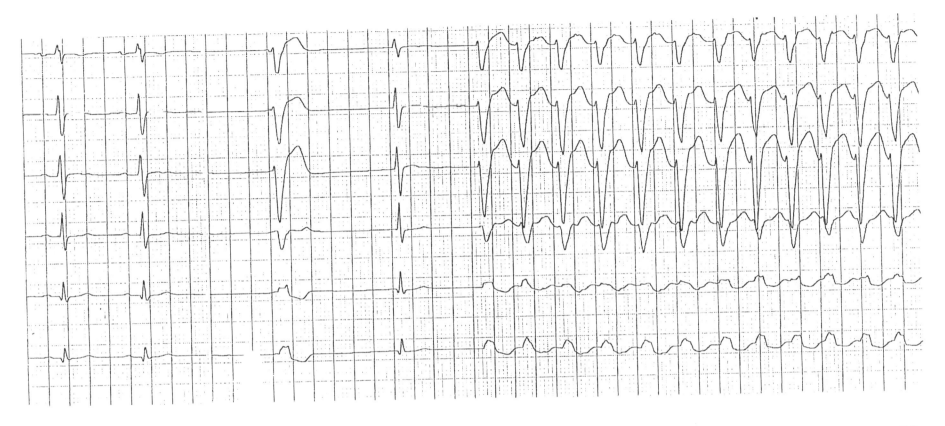

A 15-year-old student presents with a 12-year history of palpitations. They have been getting progressively worse for the past few years, lasting for several hours. While being examined in the office, the patient began to have paroxysms of tachycardia and a simultaneous 6-lead electrocardiogram was obtained. From top to bottom ECG leads are $V_1$ to $V_6$. What EP observations can be made, and what is the differential diagnosis?

*Figure 4–12B*

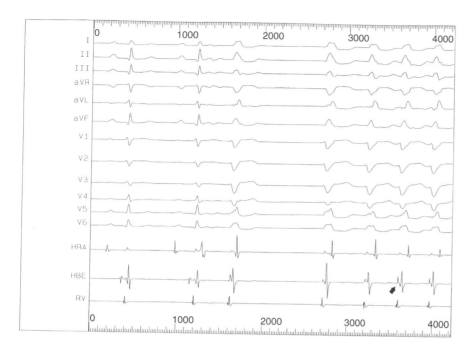

**Explanation:**

In Fig. 4–12A, the initiating and tachycardia QRS complexes appear almost identical. Since there is no atrial activity preceding the initiating beat, VT was highly suspect. The third QRS complex is similar to the tachycardia morphology and does not originate from the atrium. This also suggested the possibility of VT. However, contrary to this diagnosis is the presence of a typical LBBB morphology during tachycardia, and the presence of normal ventricular function by echocardiography. This essentially excludes bundle branch reentry, but does not exclude idiopathic septal VT. Therefore, one had to consider alternative possibilities, which were uncovered at EP study.

At EP study (Fig. 4–12B), spontaneous onset of tachycardia is remarkably similar to that noted in Fig. 4–12A. The His bundle deflection is easily identified with the first two sinus complexes. The third QRS complex is caused by a PAC and has the morphology of the tachycardia. It appears that a His bundle deflection is present within the early portion of the ventricular electrogram; retrograde atrial activity is noted. The fourth QRS complex has a similar morphology and is also associated with retrograde atrial activity, but no initial atrial activity. This is followed by the tachycardia, and the last two QRS complexes are associated with a His bundle deflection occurring shortly after activation of the ventricle (*arrow*).

This situation was clarified in Fig. 4–12C. During tachycardia a PAC was introduced in the high right atrium. The septal atrial electrogram was refractory at this time as noted on the proximal His bundle lead. However, the premature atrial complex preexcited the ventricle (376 ms on RV lead) and did so with an identical QRS complex as noted during tachycardia. This confirmed the presence of anterograde conduction over an AP (see earlier discussion). This observation was made during onset of atrial pacing during tachycardia. At other parts of the study the presence of an atriofascicular pathway was confirmed and the final diagnosis was atriofascicular reentry and not VT. Reanalysis of Fig. 4–12A suggests that the onset of tachycardia in this patient may have occurred secondary to automaticity in the atriofascicular tract. These pathways are known to have retrograde block. It is impossible to exclude a ventricular premature complex originating very close to the insertion site of the right bundle branch in this patient.

In summary, because of the extremely unusual initiation of tachycardia and the relative rarity of the phenomenon in this patient, the ECG diagnosis was more difficult than usual. One should always include atriofascicular reentry in the differential diagnosis of a typical LBBB tachycardia in a patient with normal ventricular function. This case emphasizes the need for EP evaluation in such patients.

## Figure 4–12C

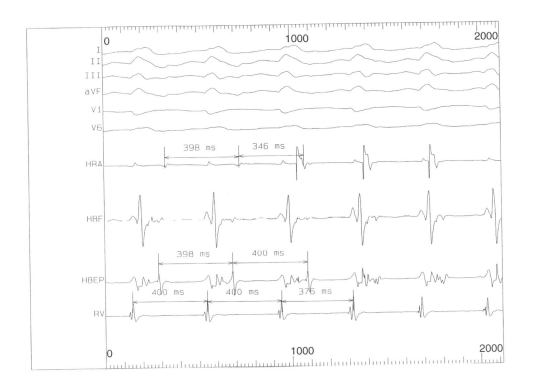

## Figure 4–13A

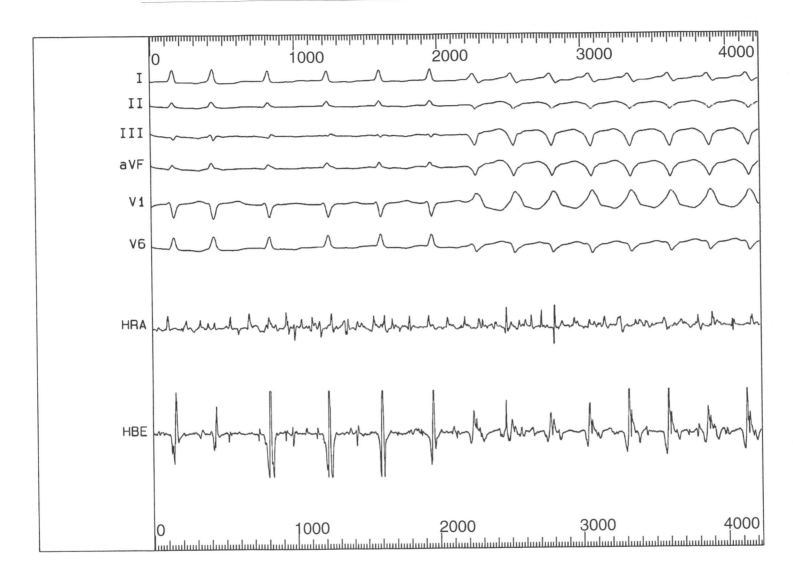

The trace shown occurred at EP study. How many tachycardias are present and what are they?

# Figure 4–13B

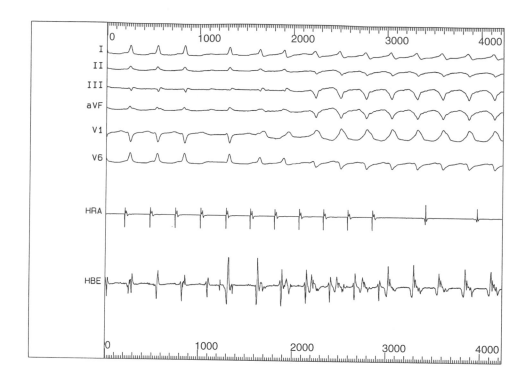

## Explanation:

In Fig. 4–13*A*, the underlying rhythm is atrial fibrillation as documented on the high right atrial recording. There are both narrow and wide QRS complexes. The narrow QRS complexes have an irregularly irregular rhythm consistent with atrial fibrillation. A His bundle electrogram is not well visualized in all complexes, but is present in several beats. The wide QRS complex tachycardia is a regular rhythm and not consistent with atrial fibrillation. Favoring VT is the appearance of the first wide QRS complex without any preceding long–short sequence, which usually occurs with aberrancy.

The RBBB morphology in $V_1$ also suggests VT, although a preexcited QRS morphology cannot be excluded. To diagnose a preexcited tachycardia one would have to suggest the very unlikely possibility of transition of atrial fibrillation to a regular tachycardia, and conduction over an AP only during the regular faster rhythm. Figure 4–13*B* shows initiation of VT with VA dissociation on the right-hand portion of the figure. Atrial pacing very infrequently induces VT. Note that VT occurs when a critical preceding ventricular rate was present, similar to what happened during atrial fibrillation. This is a very unusual variety of tachycardia-induced tachycardia (see discussion of Fig. 4–5).

## Figure 4–14A

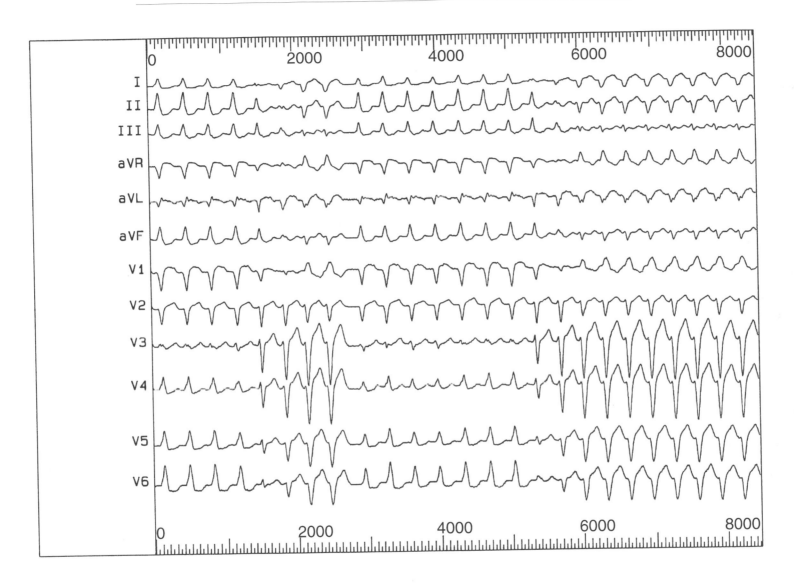

This elderly woman had a history of nonsustained wide QRS complex tachycardia and underwent EP evaluation. The simultaneous 12-lead ECG shown was recorded at EP study. What is the diagnosis?

## Figure 4–14B

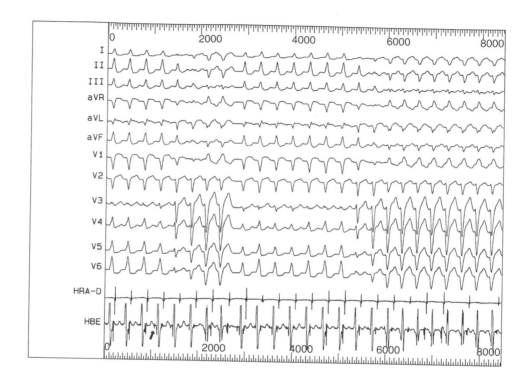

## Explanation:

The intracardiac electrograms are included in Fig. 4–14B. Narrow and wide QRS complex tachycardias are present. The first four QRS complexes are representative of the narrow QRS tachycardia, and a His bundle deflection is present before ventricular activation (*arrow*). The wide QRS tachycardia has an RBBB morphology as noted in $V_1$. Note that fusion beats occur during the transition from the narrow to wide QRS tachycardia. A His bundle deflection is not routinely present before ventricular activation in the wide complex tachycardia, which is VT. Further, after VT terminates the SVT, VA block is also present as noted at the end of the tracing. The rates of tachycardia are similar, but the wide QRS tachycardia is clearly faster. EP testing confirmed AV node reentry for the narrow QRS tachycardia. The VT typically occurred during AV node reentry and is an example of tachycardia-induced tachycardia. It usually terminated AV node reentry, but was nonsustained at all times. The VT could also occur without preceding AV node reentry and, therefore, elimination of AV node reentry would not be expected to prevent recurrences of VT in this patient.

# *Figure 4–15A*

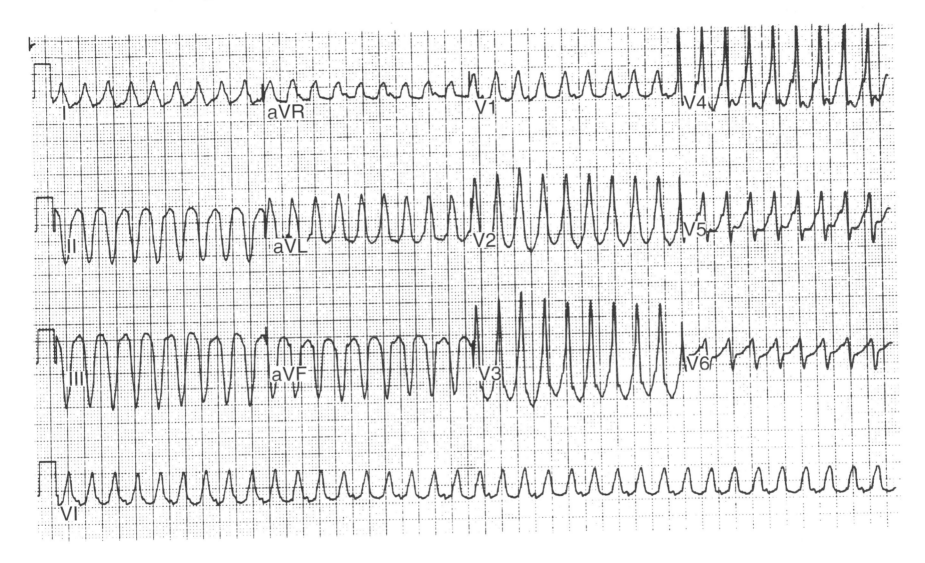

This patient presented with a history of syncope. At EP study the 12-led ECG shown was recorded. What is the most likely diagnosis?

Is antidromic tachycardia using a left free wall AP part of the differential diagnosis?

## *Figure 4–15B*

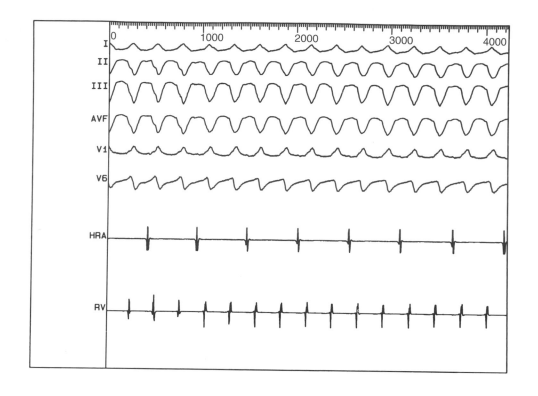

**Explanation:**

Figure 4–15*B* includes the intracardiac electrograms. Note that the RBBB tachycardia is associated with 2:1 VA conduction. In fact, this is clearly seen during careful inspection of the 12-lead ECG in Fig. 4–15*A* (lead V₁). The most likely diagnosis is VT. Antidromic tachycardia should not be considered since 1:1 VA association must be present in this situation.

## Figure 4–16A

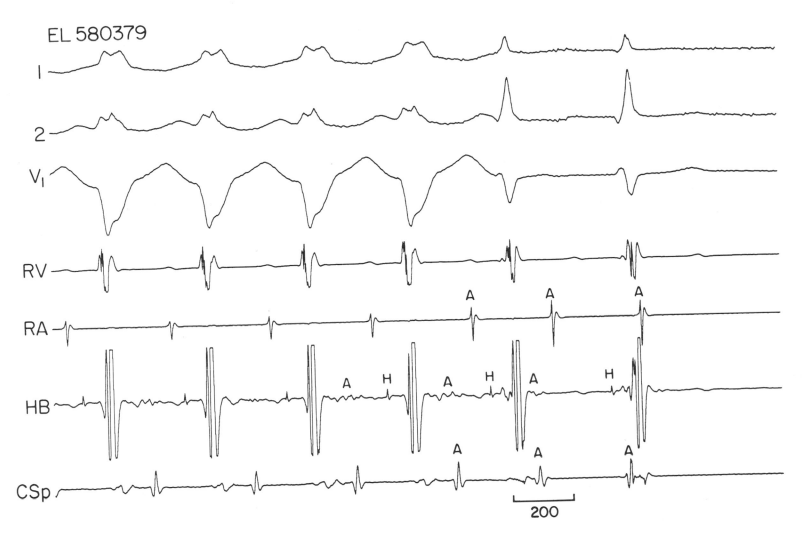

EL 580379

I

2

V₁

RV

RA

HB

CSp

200

The record is from a young patient with recurrent palpitations that always stop spontaneously after a couple of minutes. What is the tachycardia mechanism and why does it terminate spontaneously? Lead CSp is the coronary sinus electrode at the orifice of the CS.

## Figure 4–16B

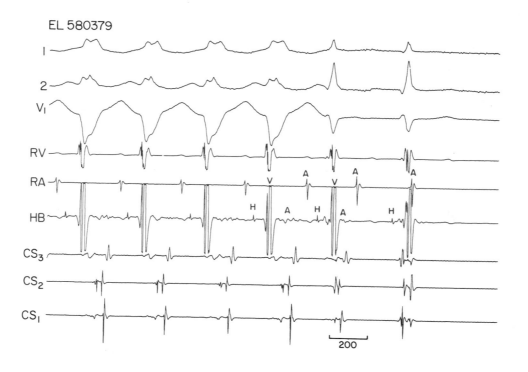

EL 580379

**Explanation:**

In essence, this wide QRS tachycardia abruptly normalizes with subsequent shortening of the VA interval (same atrial activation sequence) and blocks after the next cycle. Figure 4–16B is the same record with the addition of other CS leads with $CS_3$ at the orifice and $CS_2$ and $CS_1$, respectively, more distal. However, the diagnosis should be made readily without the additional leads. The tachycardia starts as a wide QRS tachycardia with an eccentric atrial activation sequence with earliest activation in the mid CS ($CS_2$). The typical LBBB morphology with the normal HV interval during tachycardia would favor a diagnosis of AV reentry with LBBB aberration (Chapter 1, Tables 1–7 and 1–8). The QRS abruptly normalizes with the fifth cycle with resolution of the functional LBBB during the AV reentrant tachycardia. Normalization of the QRS occurs without preceding change in the cycle length, suggesting that the mechanism of normalization is not cycle length

dependent. The mechanism is likely either progressive shortening of the left bundle branch refractory period at the newly established faster heart rate during tachycardia or sudden loss of retrograde transseptal concealed conduction into the left bundle branch. Regardless of the mechanism of normalization, it is associated with abrupt shortening of the VA interval, a reflection of the shortened tachycardia circuit resulting from elimination of transseptal conduction time from the RV to the LV. The decreased VA interval produces a shorter subsequent AA interval, which is analogous to an atrial extrastimulus or premature atrial depolarization. The "premature" atrial depolarization blocks over a fast AV node pathway and conducts over a slow AV node pathway. Tachycardia terminates spontaneously after a single AV node echo, which encounters anterograde refractoriness in the slow pathway. This is an interesting example of interplay of tachycardia mechanisms that limits rather than facilitates maintenance of tachycardia.

## *Figure 4–17A*

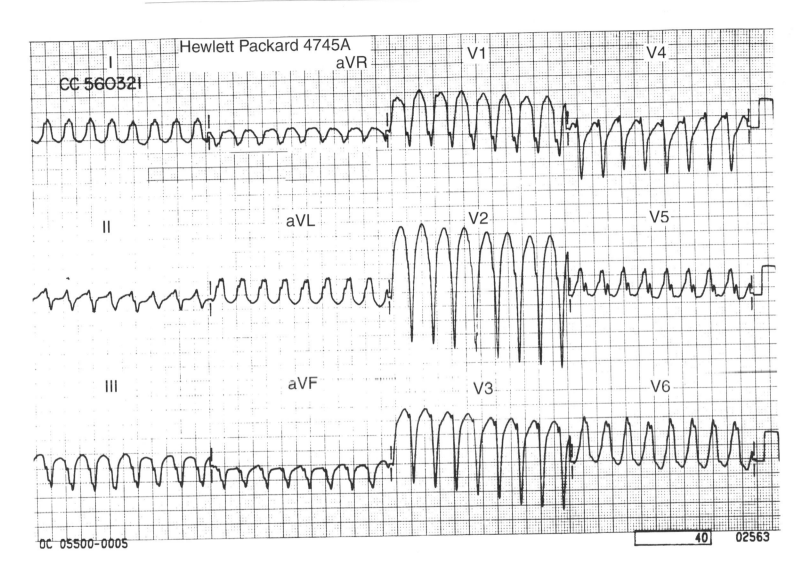

Hewlett Packard 4745A

This electrocardiogram was recorded in a 30-year-old patient with a history of tachycardia of sudden onset with no specific provocation. There was no clinical evidence of heart disease and the echocardiogram was normal. What is the mechanism of tachycardia?

# Figure 4–17B

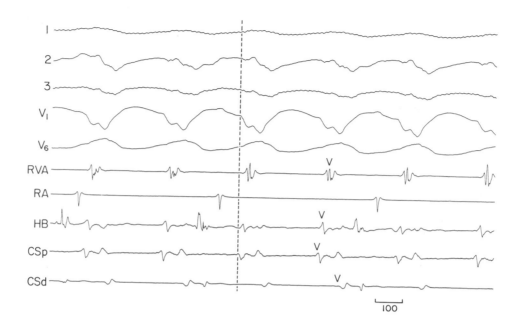

## Explanation:

The 12-lead electrocardiogram showed a regular wide QRS tachycardia with LBBB morphology. P waves were not clearly discernible. In a young patient without heart disease, a mechanism of SVT with aberration or preexcited tachycardia should be initially considered. However, this young patient clearly had VT as is evident on the intracardiac records. There was no evidence of cardiac disease in this patient after extensive investigation and this tachycardia would be classified as "idiopathic" VT. The most common type of idiopathic VT originates in the RV outflow region and is associated with LBBB and inferior axis. This morphology is unusual, suggesting an origin of VT in the "posteroseptal" region (earliest ventricular activation in Fig. 4–17B is recorded in CSp, the electrode at the orifice of the CS). LBBB morphology, especially related to areas other than the RV outflow region, should raise a suspicion of arrhythmogenic right ventricular dysplasia for which no evidence could be found in this individual.

# Figure 4–18A

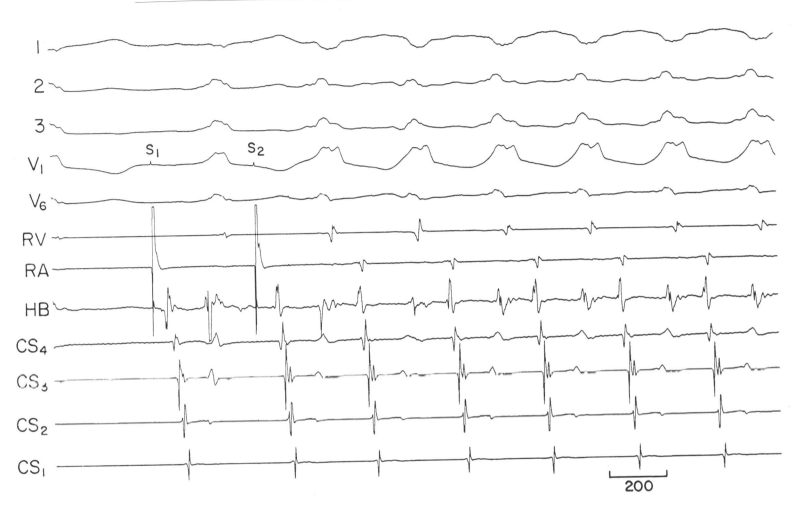

The record is from a 13-year-old boy with a history of recurrent tachycardia of sudden onset. The 12-lead electrocardiogram in sinus rhythm showed a left lateral preexcitation pattern. $CS_4$ is in the orifice of the coronary sinus and $CS_3$ to $CS_1$ are progressively more distal. $S_1$ is the last of a drive of eight right atrial paced beats at cycle length 600 ms and $S_2$ is an atrial extrastimulus. What is the mechanism of tachycardia?

## *Figure 4–18B*

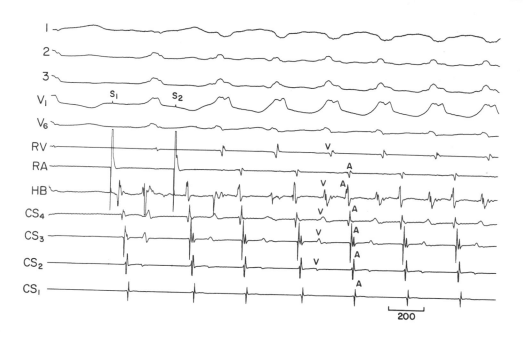

## Explanation:

The QRS morphology during established tachycardia is identical to that observed during atrial pacing and reflects conduction over a left lateral AP. Supporting this is earliest ventricular activation on the available leads at the distal CS. Atrial activation sequence begins in the His bundle region and we can therefore classify this tachycardia as a preexcited tachycardia with a concentric atrial activation sequence (Chapter 1, Table 1–9). This tracing alone does not establish whether the pathway was part of the tachycardia circuit. Both atrial tachycardia and AV node reentry were ruled out by demonstrating that relatively long coupled atrial premature extrastimuli conducted over the AP and advanced and reset tachycardia. Accepting that the AP was part of the tachycardia circuit, the major dilemma now is to determine whether the retrograde limb is the normal AV conduction system or a second retrogradely conducting septal AP. This must be established by pacing techniques, a useful one relying on the observation that PVCs delivered into tachycardia near the His bundle region will preexcite the atrium at much longer coupling intervals than pacing at the right ventricular apex when an anteroseptal pathway is the retrograde limb, and will require shorter coupling intervals when the AV node is the retrograde limb. This fundamental physiologic observation is merely based on proximity of the pacing site to the entrance of the excitable gap in the circuit. It is thus clear that the diagnostic possibilities in Chapter 1, Table 1–9, can only be distinguished in this record for certainty with dynamic observations and not from this record alone.

## *Figure 4–19A*

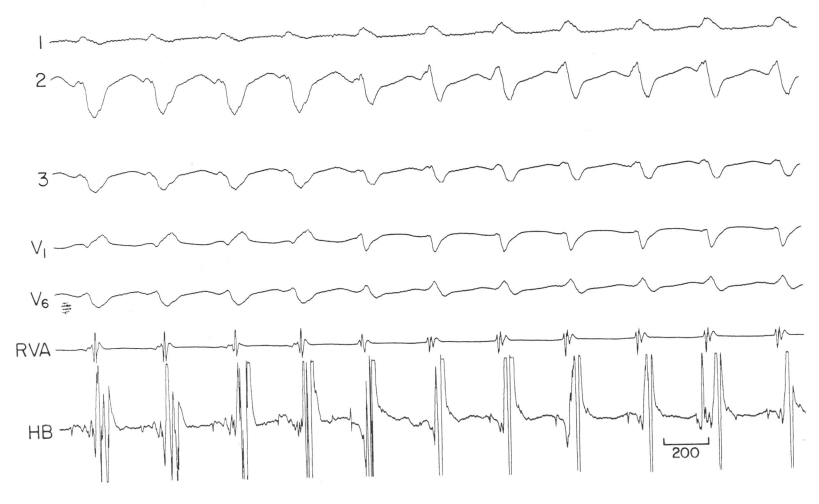

I

2

3

V₁

V₆

RVA

HB

200

The record is taken from a 73-year-old man who presented with wide QRS tachycardia several years after uncomplicated anterior MI. The tachycardia was consistently induced by two extrastimuli that resulted in prolongation of the VH interval after the extrastimu- lus. The HV during sinus rhythm was 55 ms and was approximately 40 ms during tachycardia. Will ablation of the right bundle branch cure this tachycardia?

## *Figure 4–19B*

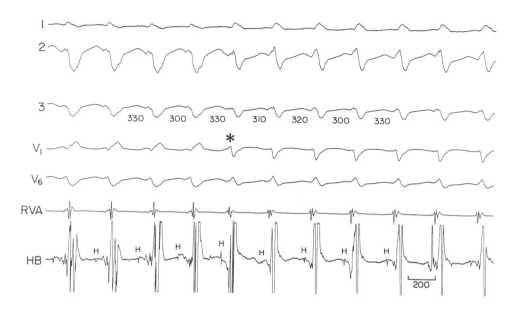

## Explanation:

The therapeutic decision is dependent on the mechanism of tachycardia. The diagnosis of VT is supported by the clinical setting and the AV dissociation evident on the His bundle channel (atrial electrogram clearly preceding next to last V). It is tempting to diagnose bundle branch reentry (see Fig. 4–10). However, a distinct change in morphology of this tachycardia from right bundle type to left bundle type is observed at the asterisk without any change in cycle length of the tachycardia or the apparent HV interval. This transition (Chapter 1, Table 1–3) is critical to mechanism as transition from right bundle to left bundle in a single cycle without change in tachycardia rate is virtually inconceivable for bundle branch reentry. Intramyocardial or distal fascicular reentry with secondary penetration of the His bundle is a much more tenable mechanism to explain this observation. This must always be considered in a situation that appears to be bundle branch reentry. Ablation of the right bundle branch will not cure this tachycardia.

## *Figure 4–20A*

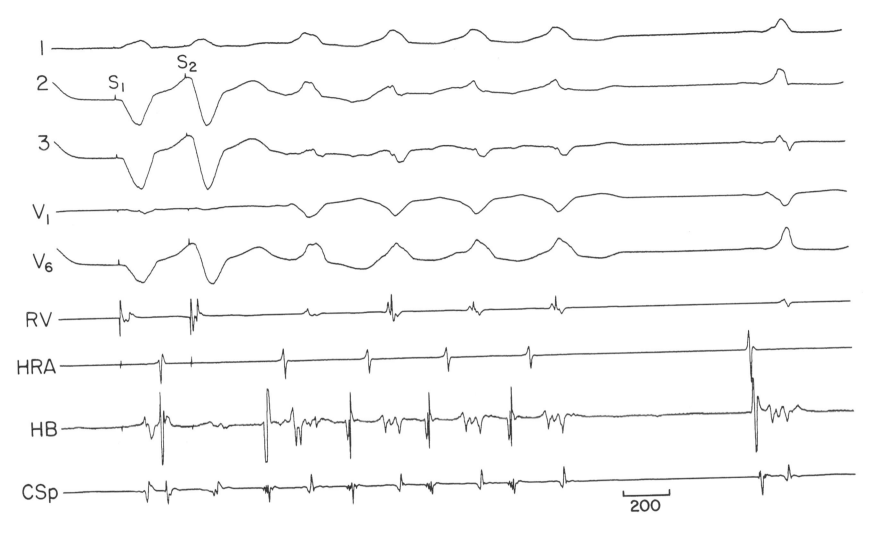

The record is taken from a young woman with a WPW pattern on the 12-lead electrocardiogram compatible with a right anteroseptal AP. $S_1$ is the last of a drive of eight ventricular cycles from the right ventricular apex at cycle length 600 ms and $S_2$ is a ventricular extrastimulus. What is the mechanism of tachycardia?

*Figure 4–20B*

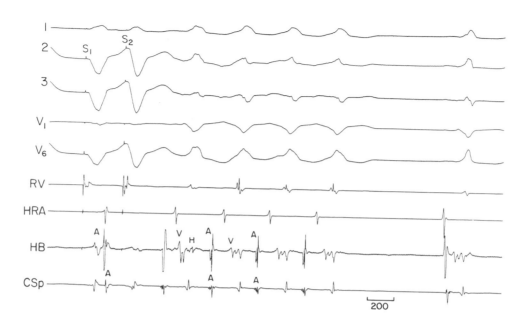

## Explanation:

This can be considered a preexcited tachycardia since there is no H preceding the QRS and the QRS morphology is compatible with the preexcitation pattern seen in sinus rhythm. The issues related to this tachycardia were discussed in the explanation section of Fig. 4–18B. In this instance, a diagnosis of nonsustained antidromic tachycardia utilizing the normal AV conduction system as the retrograde limb can be made with reasonable certainty. $S_1$ conducts over the AP with a short VA interval and $S_2$ fails to conduct over the AP. Note that a retrograde His deflection is clearly observed after the first tachycardia cycle. The His merges into the V with a second cycle (His not seen) with shortening of the VA interval and proportional advancement of the next preexcited QRS. Resolution of retrograde conduction delay in the HPS after the first cycle or two is not unusual at the onset of antidromic tachycardia.

## Figure 4–21A

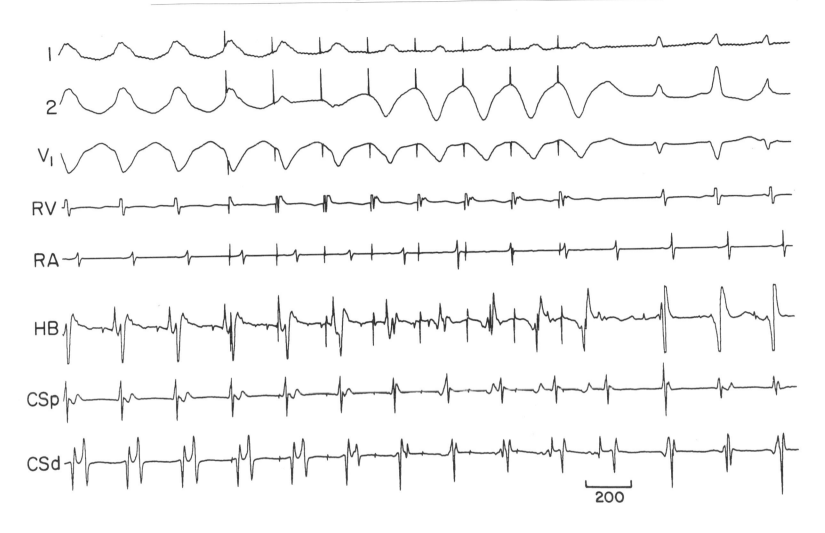

The record is from a 43-year-old woman with a history of paroxysmal tachycardia. Tachycardia of LBBB morphology was reproducibly induced by atrial extrastimuli attaining a critical AH delay. What happened after a burst of ventricular pacing was introduced into this tachycardia? CSp is the coronary sinus electrode at the orifice of the CS, and CSd is in the distal CS.

# Figure 4–21B

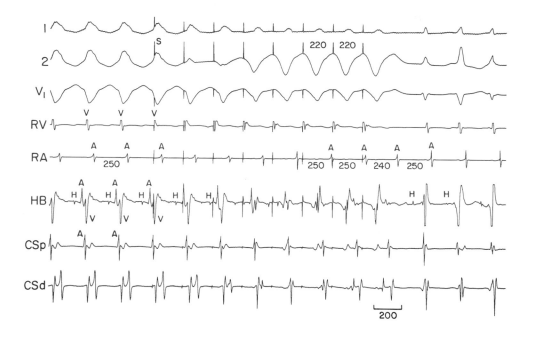

## Explanation:

The clinical and EP presentation in this patient is typical for AV node reentry. Tachycardia has a relatively short cycle length of 250 ms and it would not be unusual for acceleration-dependent LBBB to be observed in this instance. A burst of ventricular pacing at a slightly shorter cycle length (220 ms) does not perceptibly alter the tachycardia mechanism, which continues with the identical cycle length but with a normal QRS after the burst. This would suggest that the mechanism of LBBB during this tachycardia is not simply acceleration dependent but related to concealed retrograde transeptal conduction that was altered by the ventricular pacing burst.

# Figure 4-22A

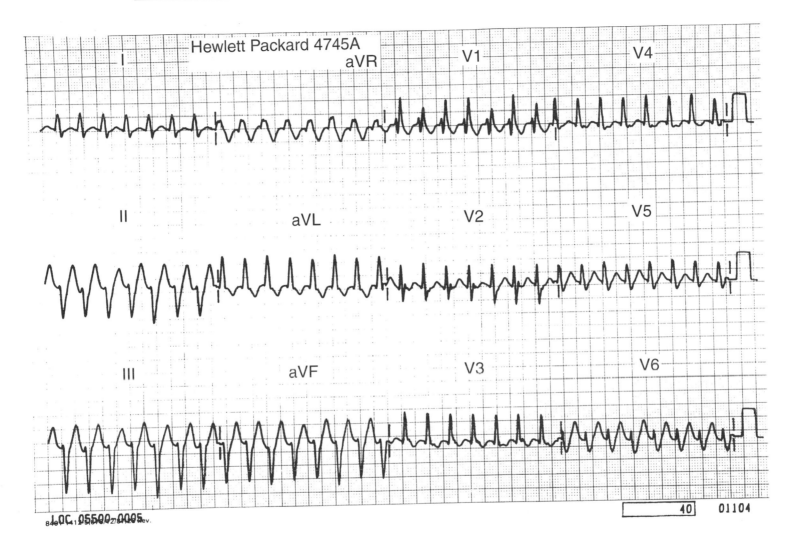

Hewlett Packard 4745A

I  aVR  V1  V4

II  aVL  V2  V5

III  aVF  V3  V6

LOC 055000 0005

40    01104

The 12-lead electrocardiogram is recorded from a patient with a long-standing history of paroxysmal, well-tolerated tachycardia frequently converted in the emergency room with intravenous verapamil. There is no associated cardiac disease. What is the differential diagnosis of this tachycardia?

# Figure 4–22B

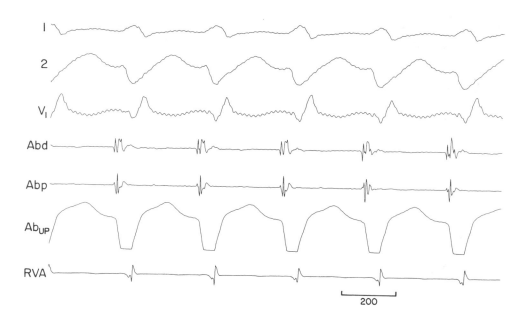

I

2

V$_1$

Abd

Abp

Ab$_{UP}$

RVA

200

## Explanation:

The clinical history and electrocardiogram would immediately suggest a diagnosis of paroxysmal SVT with aberrant conduction. There are, however, electrocardiographic features that do not support this diagnosis. First, the RBBB pattern is slightly atypical with a deep S wave in V$_6$. Secondly, there is striking left axis deviation in addition to the RBBB aberration, a pattern of bifascicular block that is distinctly unusual in paroxysmal SVT. Finally, there is a suggestion of AV dissociation best appreciated in lead V$_3$. This is a very typical electro-

cardiogram for patients with the most common type of idiopathic left VT (verapamil-sensitive VT). This tachycardia is believed to originate from reentry in the distal Purkinje system in the left ventricular apical-septal region. The intracardiac record in Fig. 4–22B demonstrates a catheter (Abd) at the site of earliest ventricular activation during tachycardia recording a typical Purkinje-type spike preceding the QRS. The recording was made prior to successful ablation of tachycardia at this site. Abd, Abp, and Ab$_{up}$ represent the distal, proximal and unipolar distal poles of the ablation catheter, respectively. RVA is the right ventricular apex.

## *Figure 4-23A*

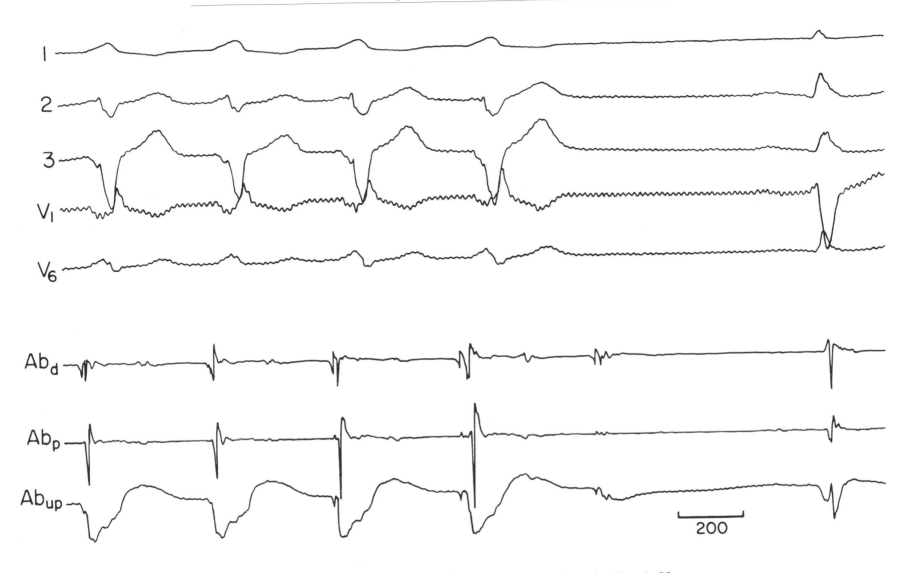

This intracardiac record is recorded from the patient in Fig. 4–22 with mapping in the region of interest described in Fig. 4–22B. What has happened?

# Figure 4–23B

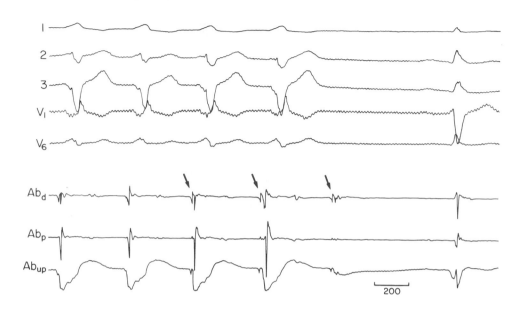

## Explanation:

This tachycardia terminated during catheter manipulation in the region recording earliest ventricular activation during tachycardia preceded by the Purkinje spike (*arrows*). This tachycardia terminated spontaneously on several occasions during such maneuvering, probably due to catheter pressure in a region critical for sustaining tachycardia ("bump mapping"). The record would suggest that termination of tachycardia was related to conduction block between the Purkinje spike and the QRS.

# Figure 4–24A

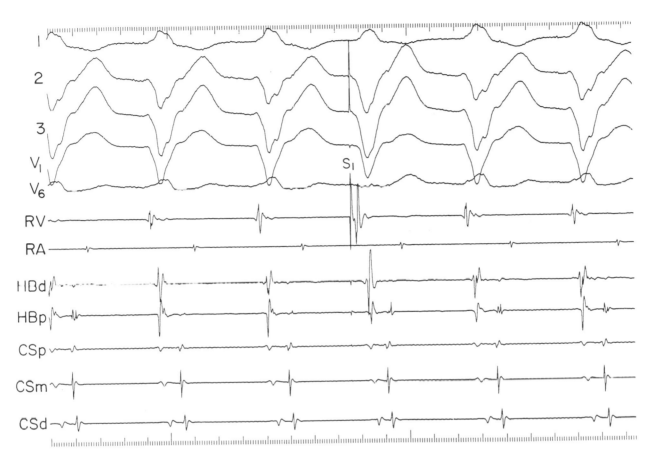

The intracardiac records are from a young woman without heart disease and a history of paroxysmal tachycardia. EP testing prior to tachycardia induction revealed a decremental, right free wall accessory AV pathway with the maximal preexcited morphology observed during atrial pacing identical to that observed in the recorded tachycardia in the figure. What is learned from the ventricular extrastimulus ($S_1$) delivered from the right ventricular apical region? HBd and HBp are His bundle records from the distal and proximal recording electrodes, respectively. CSp, CSm, and CSd represent coronary sinus recordings from the proximal to distal coronary sinus regions, respectively, with CSp near the orifice.

# Figure 4-24B

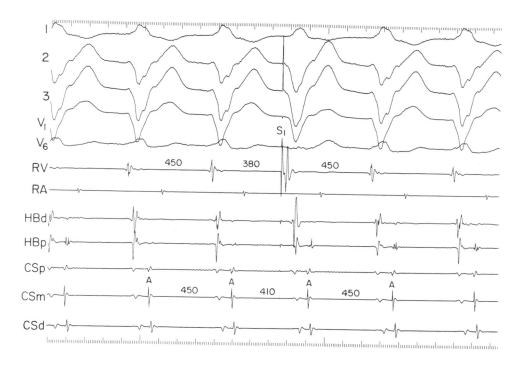

## Explanation:

Since the tachycardia has the preexcited morphology observed during atrial pacing and no preceding His deflection, it can be considered to be a preexcited tachycardia. The atrial activation sequence is concentric (Chapter 1, Tables 1–6 and 1–9). A relatively late coupled PVC preexcites the atrium and resets the tachycardia. This virtually proves that the accessory pathway is part of the tachycardia circuit (Chapter 1, Table 1–9), leaving us to determine if the retrograde atrial activation is related to the normal AV conduction system (typical antidromic tachycardia) or to a second AP in the septal region. Preexcitation from the right ventricular apical region at such a long coupling interval demonstrates excellent access to the excitable gap of the reentrant circuit which would be expected if the retrograde limb were the right bundle branch and the normal AV conduction system as was the case in this example. When the latency time after the extrastimulus is accounted for, the RV apical electrogram is advanced by only 40 ms and advances the subsequent A by 40 ms. This suggests that the RV apical electrogram is right in the circuit, which would not be the case if the retrograde limb were a second septal AP. A more definitive distinction could be made with reasonable certainty by comparing PVCs inserted into the tachycardia circuit at a right ventricular basal site near the septum versus a right ventricular apical site to determine which has easier access to the excitable gap. Theoretically, the tracing could also be explained by retrograde conduction over a nodofascicular pathway with retrograde conduction, probably a very rare entity.

# Figure 4–25A

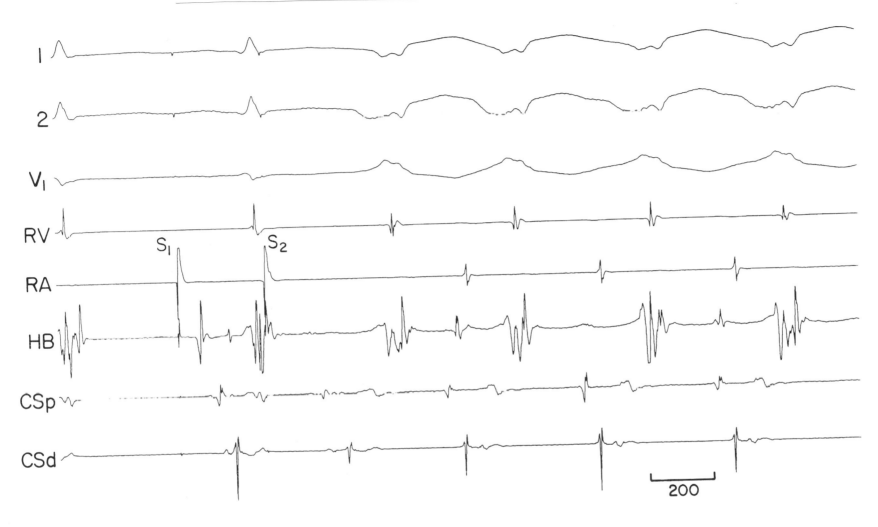

The patient is a young man with paroxysmal tachycardia in the absence of heart disease. The 12-lead electrocardiogram was normal. A wide QRS tachycardia was induced after a critically timed atrial extrastimulus as illustrated in this figure. At longer coupling intervals, the QRS was normal. What are the components of this tachycardia circuit? $S_1$ is the last of a drive of eight atrial depolarizations delivered at the high right atrium and $S_2$ is the atrial extrastimulus.

# Figure 4–25B

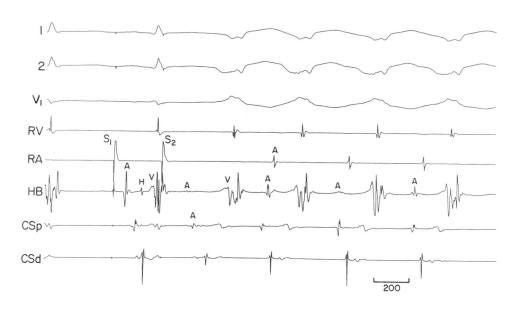

**Explanation:**

This method of induction was highly reproducible with a stable His recording site. With no H preceding the QRS (Chapter 1, Table 1–8), this can be considered to be a preexcited tachycardia. The QRS morphology could be reproduced by atrial pacing at rapid rates. VT induction by atrial extrastimuli has been described, especially in idiopathic LV VT, but one would not expect reproduction of the tachycardia QRS morphology by rapid atrial pacing in such a circumstance. Further, the $S_2$ would have to reach the ventricle before starting VT. The preexcited morphology suggests a left lateral or posterolateral AP as is supported by early ventricular activation at the distal CS electrogram (CSd). The AP has a long conduction time, a phenomenon usually observed with posteroseptal APs but also observed elsewhere. The retrograde limb of this tachycardia has a concentric atrial activation sequence with atrial activation occurring first at the orifice of the coronary sinus (CSp) slightly ahead of the His bundle electrogram. As discussed previously (Chapter 1, Table 1–9, and Fig. 4–24) we must distinguish retrograde conduction occurring over the AV node versus over a septal AP. In this particular instance, retrograde conduction proceeded over a slow AV node pathway, as could be demonstrated by inserting PVCs into the cardiac cycle during tachycardia. Preexcitation from the right ventricular apical region would preexcite the atria at a relatively longer coupling interval than PVCs from the base of the heart near the AP, demonstrating better access to the excitable gap of the reentrant circuit, which would be expected if the retrograde limb were the right bundle branch and the normal AV conduction system (see Fig. 4–24). This antidromic tachycardia is unusual in that the AP has a long anterograde conduction time and retrograde conduction was proceeding over a slow AV node pathway.

# *Figure 4–26A*

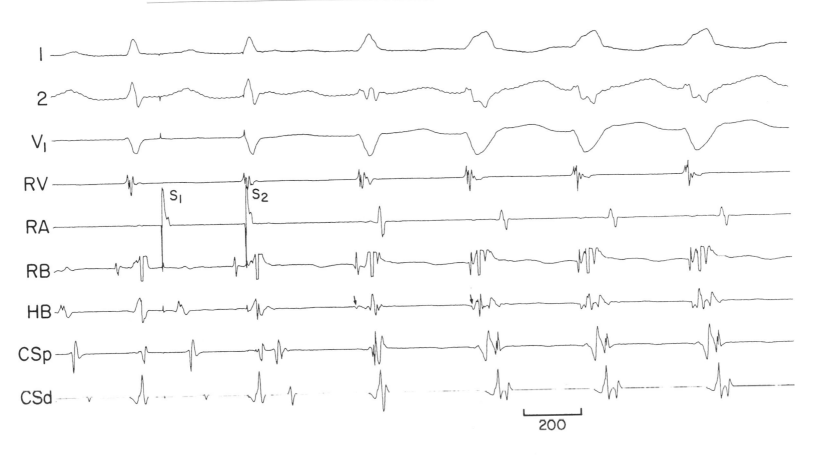

The patient is a 15-year-old boy with a recent history of paroxysmal tachycardia, no heart disease, and a normal 12-lead electrocardiogram. At EP testing, incremental atrial pacing from the lateral right atrium resulted in a preexcited QRS morphology that was not observed during similar atrial pacing from the proximal CS. The A to preexcited QRS conduction time was long. Wide QRS tachycardia with identical morphology to the preexcited QRS was initiated with a critically timed atrial extrastimulus as shown in the record. What are the observations? CSp and CSd are recorded from the proximal and distal coronary sinus, respectively, with the proximal recording near the orifice of the CS. HB and RB are at right bundle branch and His bundle recording sites.

# Figure 4–26B

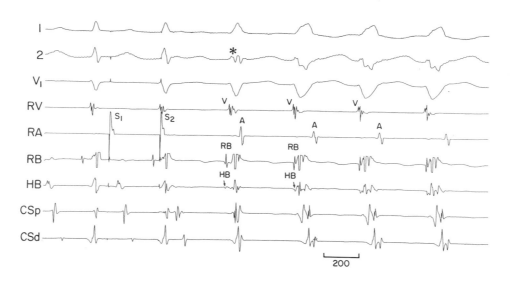

## Explanation:

The preceding description and the QRS morphology during the preexcited tachycardia suggest a right-sided AP with a long conduction time ("decremental"). The rapid component of the right ventricular electrogram at the right ventricular apex is approximately at the onset of the QRS, an observation compatible with an atriofascicular AP that activates the right ventricle near the right bundle branch terminus, as was the case in this patient. Note also that the right bundle electrogram during tachycardia is also at the onset of the QRS and precedes activation of the His bundle (less well seen) by 5 to 10 ms. We are then left with a preexcited tachycardia (over a right atriofascicular pathway) with retrograde activation of the right bundle branch and, subsequently, the His bundle. The atrial activation sequence is concentric and is probably proceeding over the normal AV conduction system. However, this can only be determined with certainty by other measures such as the relative ability of PVCs from the right ventricular apical region and the base of the heart near the His bundle to preexcite the atrium during tachycardia. In this differential diagnosis, remember that the most common regular preexcited tachycardia (that is excluding atrial fibrillation) is true antidromic tachycardia with conduction over the AP and a return circuit via the normal AV conduction system. An astute observer will also notice that the first tachycardia cycle (asterisk) is a little different from the subsequent cycles with the QRS being a reasonable fusion between the normal QRS and the totally preexcited QRS. Furthermore, the His bundle electrogram (low amplitude) *precedes* the right bundle by a few milliseconds, supporting the view that the tachycardia has not yet started at this point since the AV node has been activated anterogradely. In fact, antegrade conduction is proceeding over a slow AV node pathway that is associated with an AV node echo cycle over a retrograde fast AV node pathway, which subsequently results in a fully preexcited QRS and the beginning of antidromic reentry. Although antidromic tachycardia is the most common tachycardia with atriofascicular APs, there is an association with AV node reentry and, indeed, other APs.

## Figure 4–27A

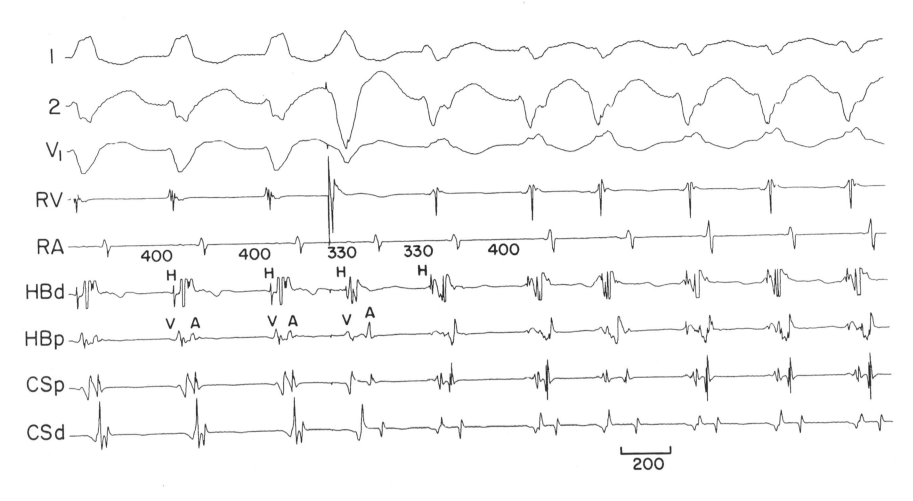

The record is from the patient described in Fig. 4–26. A PVC is introduced into the cardiac cycle during the antidromic tachycardia described in the previous case. What observations can be made from this "zone of transition"? HBd and HBp are recordings from the proximal and distal electrodes of a standard His bundle catheter (bipolar recordings, four poles, 10-mm separation). CSp and CSd are proximal and distal coronary sinus electrodes, respectively, with the proximal electrode being near the orifice of the CS.

# Figure 4–27B

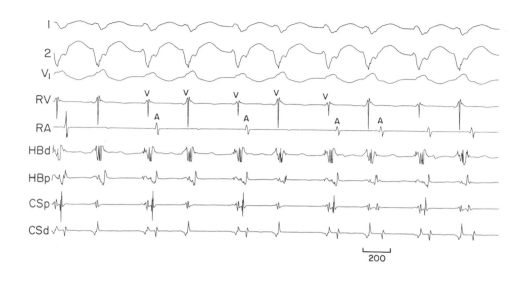

## Explanation:

The right ventricular apical extrastimulus readily preexcites both His and atrial activation without changing atrial activation sequence, an observation compatible with antidromic reentry with a relatively large excitable gap accessible to the right ventricular apical catheter by virtue of its proximity to the distal right bundle branch. This is not unexpected. However, there is a change in QRS morphology after the extrastimulus (now right bundle, leftward axis) and the tachycardia becomes somewhat irregular. The retrograde atrial activation sequence has not changed appreciably. The His bundle elec- trogram cannot be discerned with certainty but is probably within the QRS and certainly past the onset of the QRS. Since the His recording site was stable, this can only be VT or a preexcited tachy- cardia from a second AP. The diagnosis becomes more evident in Fig. 4–27B when the tachycardia continues in the presence of VA block, a situation not compatible with AV reentry although theoreti- cally compatible with nodoventricular or nodofascicular reentry. In this instance, this patient also had inducible idiopathic LV VT, a tachycardia never previously documented clinically in this patient. Although common things are common, it is important to be methodi- cal and continue to have an open mind and "expect the unexpected."

# Chapter 5

# Catheter Ablation

## Figure 5–1A

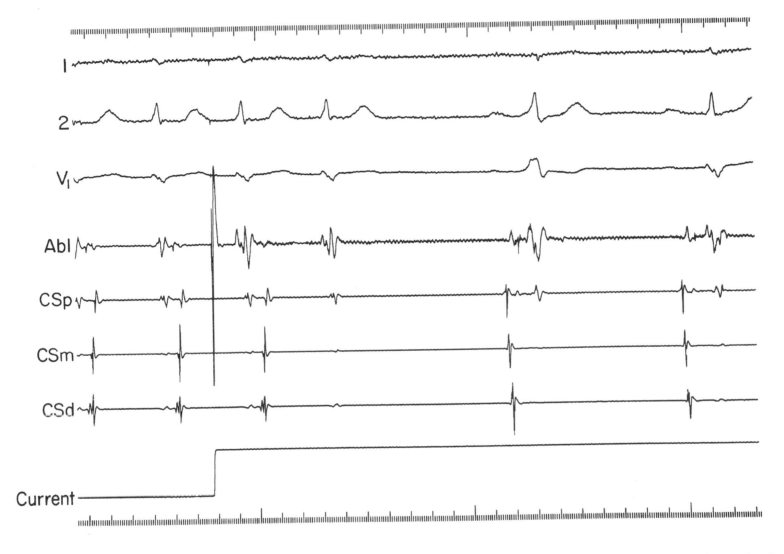

The patient is undergoing ablation of a left AP during ongoing AV reentrant tachycardia. How many accessory pathways are involved?

CSp, CSm, and Csd represent coronary sinus electrodes from CS os to distal CS positions, respectively.

# Figure 5–1B

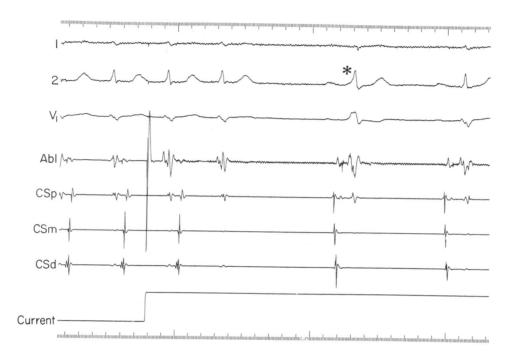

## Explanation:

Tachycardia stops within two cycles after current is applied with block occurring in the AP. However, the first sinus escape cycle is associated with a preexcited QRS (denoted by the asterisk, *) with a left lateral preexcitation pattern. Retrograde conduction has been apparently ablated prior to anterograde conduction. There are several potential explanations for this. It is indeed possible that there were two closely spaced APs with initial ablation of the one responsi-ble for retrograde conduction and the second for anterograde conduction. Alternatively, there may be longitudinal dissociation in a single fiber with the ablation injury originally sustained by the portion responsible for retrograde conduction. It may just be that the injury prolonged retrograde refractoriness to a point permitting termination of tachycardia with complete destruction of the pathway requiring a little more time. Finally, one cannot rule out a catheter-induced PVC occurring with the relative pause after termination of tachy-cardia.

## Figure 5–2A

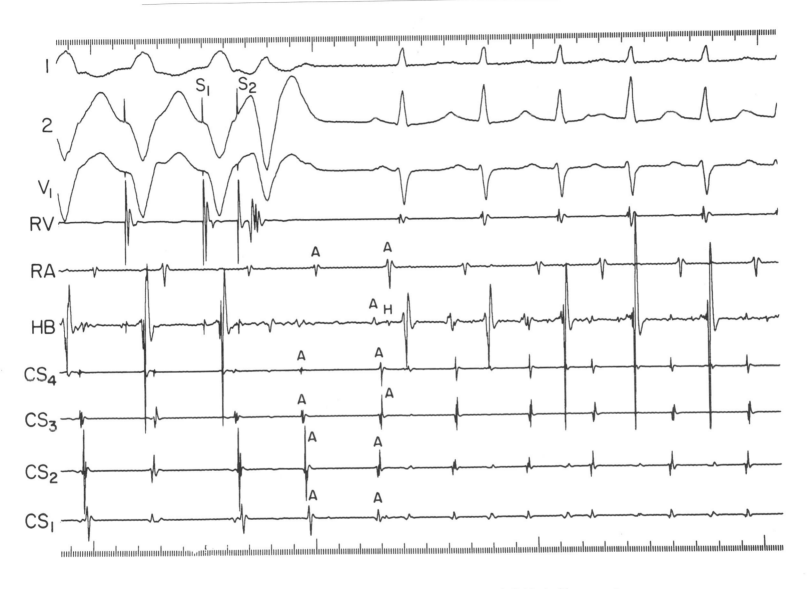

Where would one ablate this tachycardia recorded from a young individual with recurrent, paroxysmal tachycardia in the absence of preexcitation?

# Figure 5–2B

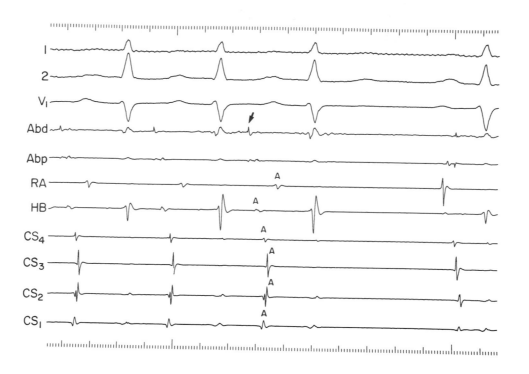

## Explanation:

The record is most consistent with an atrial tachycardia (Chapter 1, Table 1–7). The atrial activation sequence is abnormal and the first atrial activation related to tachycardia is not preceded by ventricular activation. In addition, the "apparent" VA conduction time is variable, whereas the AV conduction time is relatively constant. The atrial activation times at all the CS sites and the His bundle site are relatively close together and certainly not compatible with a single focal origin at the AV ring. In fact, the similarity of activation times at all recorded CS sites and the His bundle site would suggest that the focus is relatively equidistant from all of these sites, as indeed it was, in the roof of the left atrium. Ablation directed at the electrogram indicated (*arrow*) was successful.

## Figure 5–3A

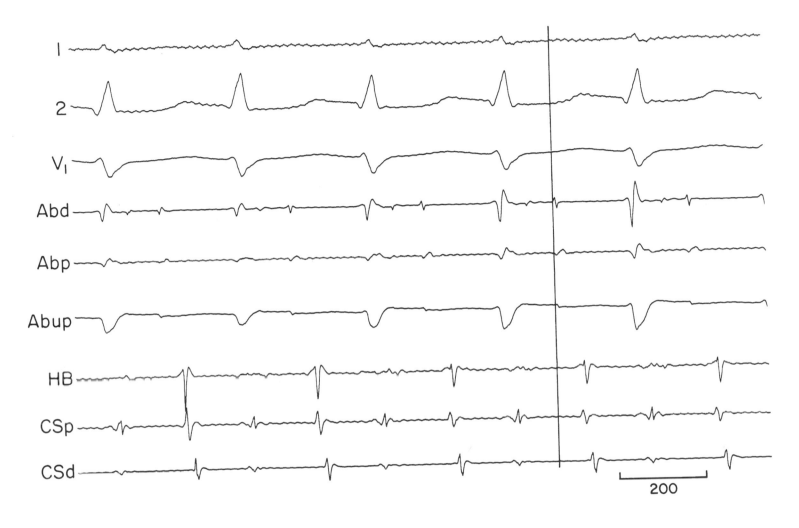

The record was from an individual otherwise well except for paroxysmal tachycardia. The tachycardia could be induced by rapid atrial pacing and extrastimuli although induction at any given rate or coupling interval was poorly reproducible. Would the site indicated be acceptable for ablation? Abd, distal electrode pair of ablation catheter; Abp, proximal pair; Abup, distal unipolar electrode.

## Figure 5–3B

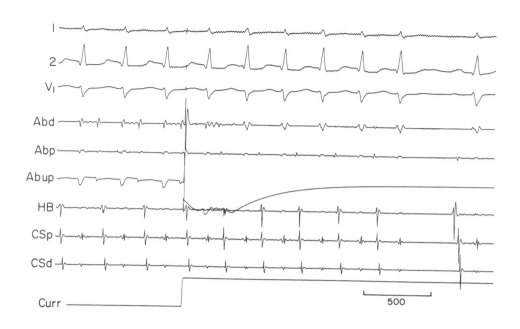

**Explanation:**

In the absence of a global atrial activation map, it is difficult to know exactly how early the earliest atrial activation during tachycardia should be. The surface P wave does give some guide if clearly seen. One can usually program PVCs into the cardiac cycle during tachycardia with the intention of advancing the QRS and exposing atrial activity without altering the atrial activation sequence. The unipolar electrogram may be helpful because this records both far-field and near-field activity. A rapid, "sharp" QS deflection at the unipolar electrogram indicates that activation is proceeding from that site and is a favorable observation. In this instance, there is no positive initial deflection in the unipolar electrogram (Abup) but there does appear to be a short isoelectric component. Nonetheless, a clear spike almost midway between ventricular and atrial activation at the ablation catheter prompted an attempt at ablation at this left atrial appendage site and was successful.

## *Figure 5–4A*

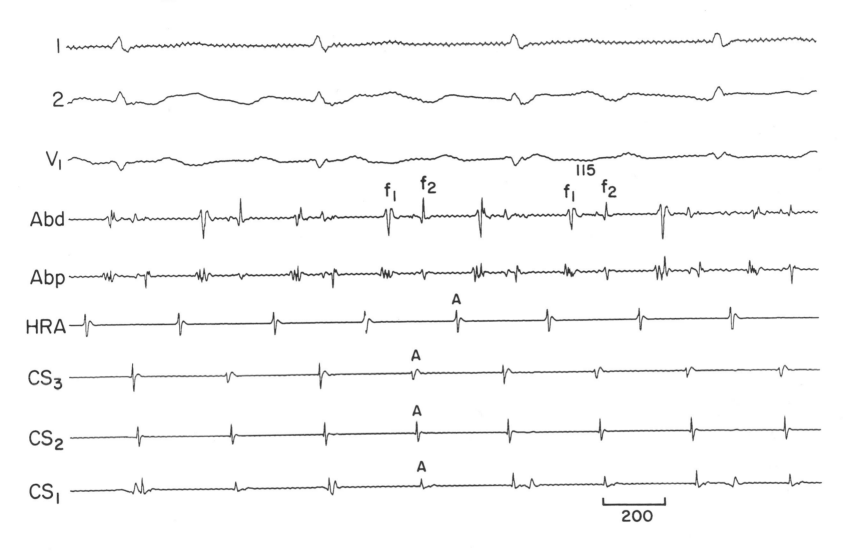

The tracing was recorded from a middle-aged patient undergoing ablation for "typical" atrial flutter. The ablation catheter is located inferior to the CS os, near the isthmus between the tricuspid valve and the inferior vena cava. What is the significance of the double activation ($f_1$, $f_2$) recorded from the ablation catheter?

# Figure 5–4B

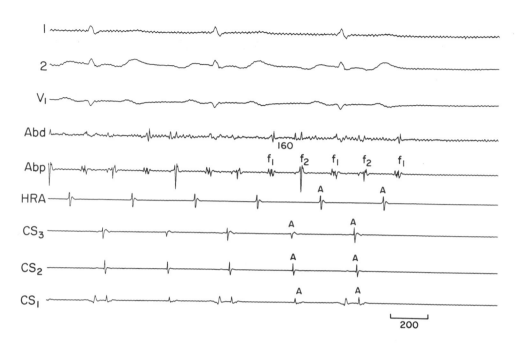

## Explanation:

These two very distinct potentials ($f_1$, $f_2$) are separated by 115 ms and suggest that the catheter is within a zone of slow conduction with the two activations representing entry ($f_1$) and exit ($f_2$) from the zone of slow conduction. Alternatively, the catheter could be straddling a line of block and recording activation on each side of the line of block but not necessarily located in a zone critical to perpetuation of reentry. In this instance, application of current at that site resulted in prolongation of the interval between $f_1$ and $f_2$ with termination of tachycardia after $f_1$. This would suggest, in retrospect, that the site was a critical zone of slow conduction with $f_1$ proximal to it and $f_2$ distal to it. It is, of course, not necessary to demonstrate this phenomenon for successful ablation.

# Figure 5–5A

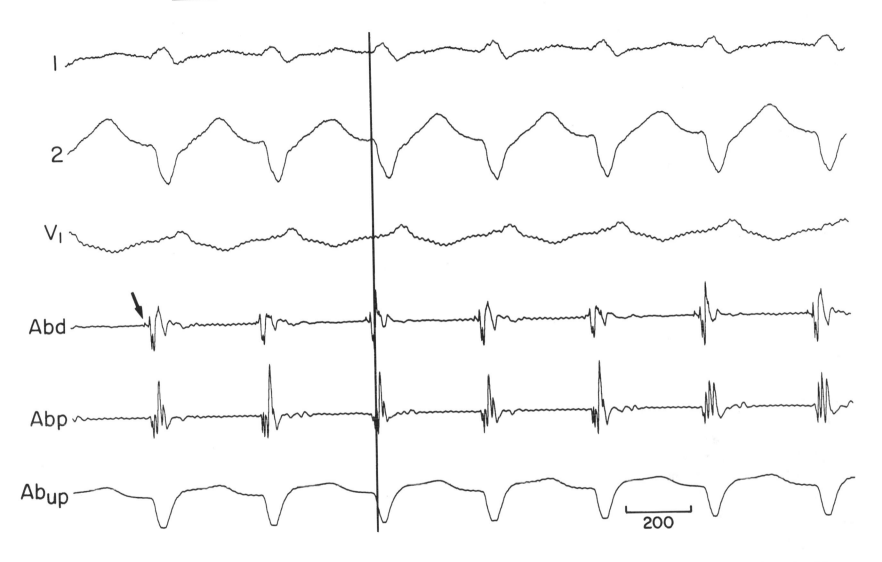

I

2

V$_1$

Abd

Abp

Ab$_{up}$

200

The record was taken during an ablation session in a patient with idiopathic left ventricular tachycardia (Belhassen type) with the abla- tion catheter located in the apical, septal region. Is this a good ablation site?

# Figure 5–5B

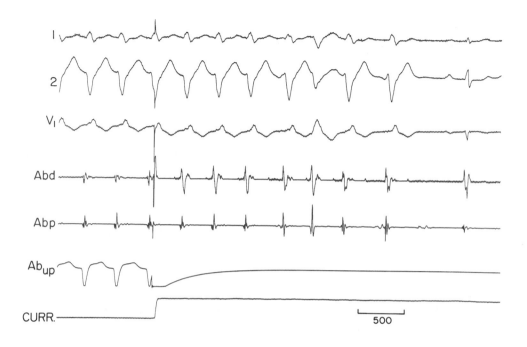

## Explanation:

Although the mechanism is still controversial, this type of tachycardia appears to have a focal origin and involve the distal Purkinje system. Ventricular activation at the successful site should precede the onset of ventricular activation on the surface QRS by at least 10 ms or more. In addition, a rapid Purkinje spike can frequently be recorded prior to ventricular activation see (*arrow*, Fig. 5–5A). The unipolar component of the ablation electrode should have a rapid and down-sloping QS deflection without initial positivity, supporting the origin of depolarization from a relative point source at the ablation catheter. Ablation at this site (30 W) was followed immediately by a slight slowing and irregularity of tachycardia prior to termination at 5 seconds.

# Figure 5–6A

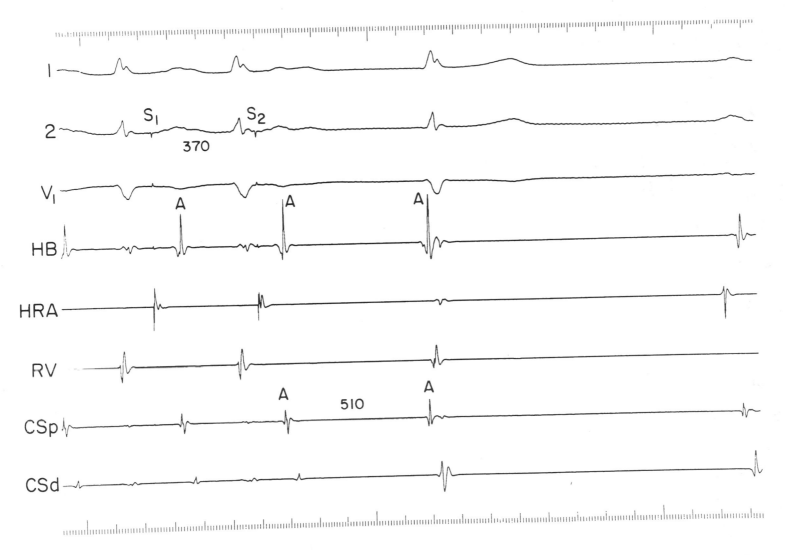

This patient had readily inducible AV node reentry (typical) prior to ablation in the "slow pathway zone" at the tricuspid annulus anterior to the CS os with this phenomenon observed after ablation. What is its significance?

# *Figure 5–6B*

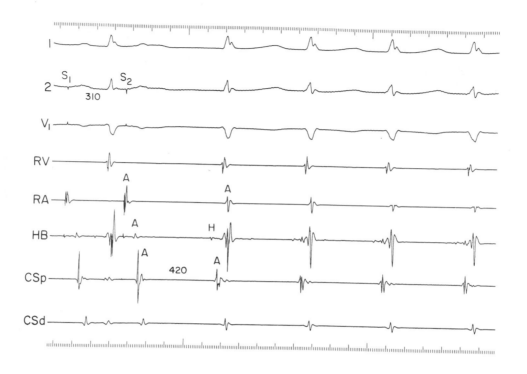

## Explanation:

The phenomenon in the record was reproducible and indicates residual slow pathway conduction associated with an AV node echo. Although elimination of slow pathway conduction is a clear and useful end point, it is not required for a successful clinical result. The addition of isoproterenol in such an example might be useful to test the integrity of the total circuit and see if sustained tachycardia can be induced. Examination of the *preablation* induction (see Fig. 5–6B) shows that the clinically documented tachycardia was induced by an extrastimulus that resulted in an interatrial interval of 420 ms measured at the proximal CS and this was the cycle length of tachycardia. After ablation, however, this interval prolonged to 510 ms. This would suggest that conduction now occurs over a second, slower pathway that may be incapable of sustained reentry or, alternatively, sufficient damage to the previous slow pathway has occurred to achieve the same result. This residual slow pathway conduction may be clinically irrelevant.

*Figure 5–7A*

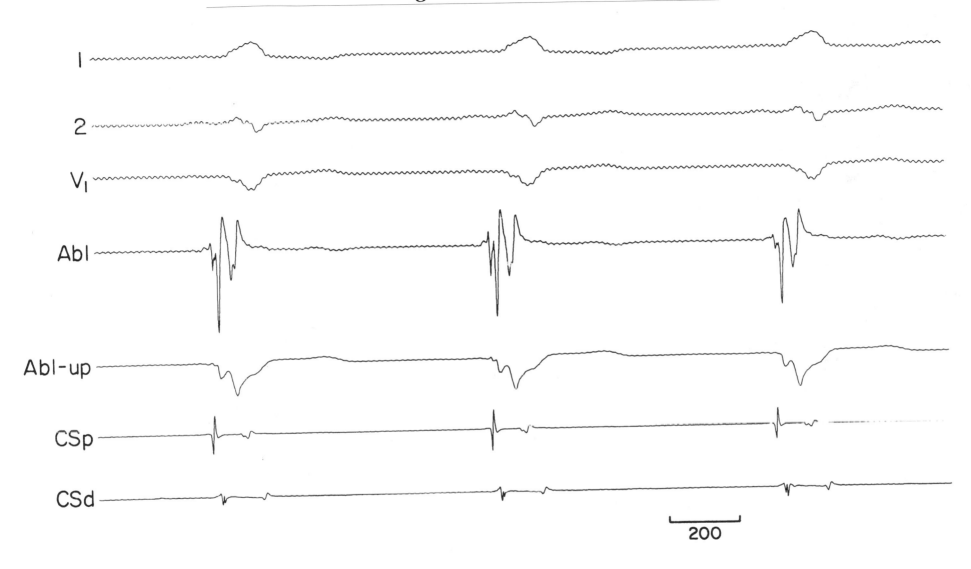

I

2

V<sub>1</sub>

Abl

Abl-up

CSp

CSd

200

The tracing was recorded from a patient with a posteroseptal preexcitation pattern who was undergoing ablation. The ablation catheter is recording from the origin of the middle cardiac vein. What does the electrogram demonstrate?

# Figure 5-7B

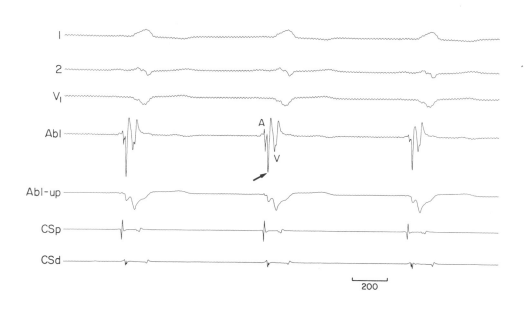

**Explanation:**

The electrogram is triphasic with the largest component being the middle component (*arrow*), which we interpreted as an AP potential. Electrograms in this region (within the coronary venous system) not infrequently have accessory pathway potentials larger than either the atrial or ventricular components. This could be verified by the extrastimulus technique, demonstrating that the AP potential does not belong to either the A or the V. For example, consider an atrial extrastimulus that results in block over the AP. Loss of the putative AP potential without change in the atrial electrogram clearly indicates that the potential in question was not part of the atrial electrogram. This was not done in this instance but the site was a successful one.

## Figure 5–8A

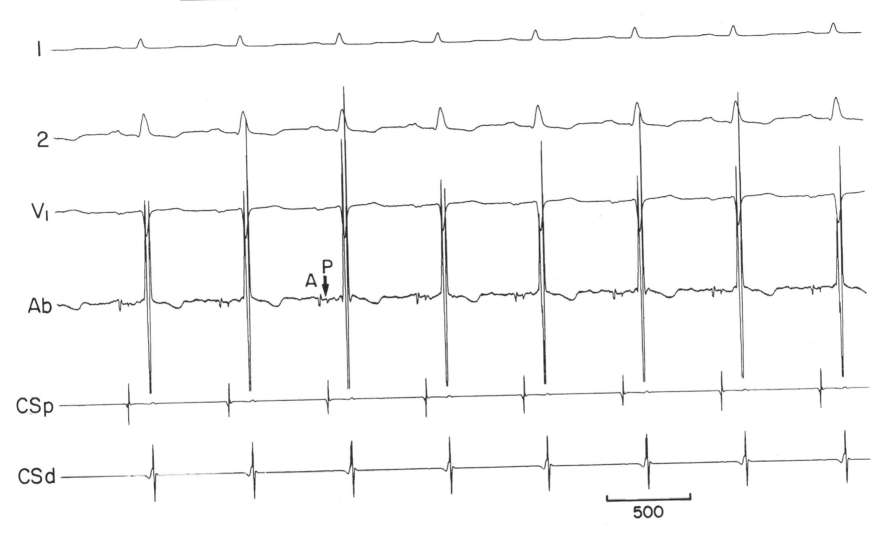

The electrogram at the ablation catheter (AB) was recorded on the tricuspid AV ring (subvalvular approach) at approximately 9 o'clock as viewed in the left anterior oblique (LAO) projection. The patient presented with antidromic tachycardia related to an atriofascicular pathway. Is this the best "target" for ablation?

# Figure 5–8B

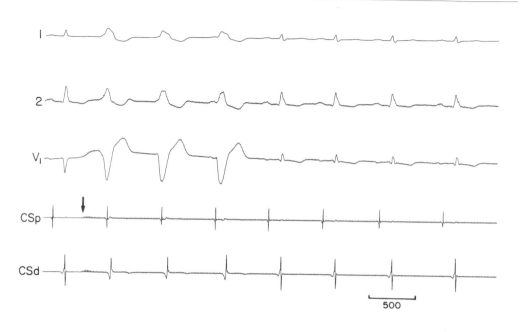

500

## Explanation:

The optimum target site for ablation of atriofascicular pathways can be problematic. Mapping of earliest ventricular activation at the AV ring is not useful since the ventricular insertion site is well within the right ventricle, near the right bundle branch (RBB) terminus. Mapping retrograde atrial activation is not useful since such pathways rarely (never?) exhibit retrograde conduction. Pacing the AV ring to find the site of pacing that gives the shortest AV conduction time has been used but is problematic in its resolution and the fact that the pathway is decremental with variability in AV conduction time.

Thus, location of the pathway potential in this particular entity at the AV ring is by far the most useful means of obtaining an appropriate target for ablation. This potential can actually be tracked through the right ventricle to its insertion site but this is technically very difficult. At this successful site, turning on current (*arrow*) immediately results in accelerated rhythm with the patient's preexcited morphology that undoubtedly represents the response of this pathway to injury. This is reminiscent of the junctional tachycardia that is seen during ablation for AV node reentry in the region of Koch's triangle and is consistent with the speculation that these are AV nodelike structures.

# Figure 5–9A

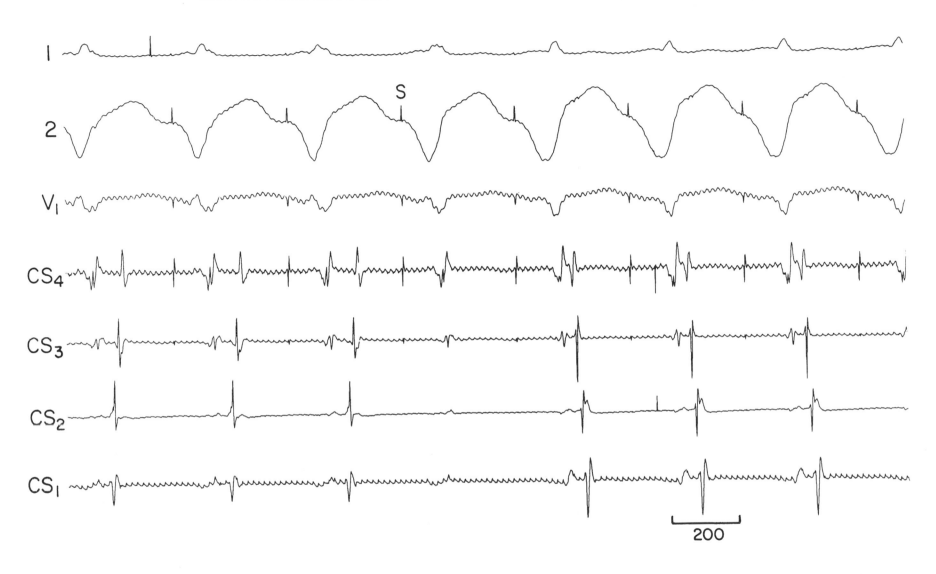

The patient was undergoing ablation of a left lateral pathway with unidirectional retrograde conduction. The decision was made to ablate during entrainment of AV reentrant tachycardia. How does one explain the sequence of events?

# Figure 5-9B

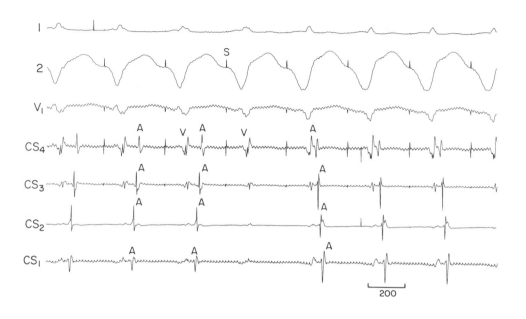

## Explanation:

Ablation during tachycardia can be problematic because sudden cessation of tachycardia with conduction block over a pathway can result in catheter movement. At times, ablation during tachycardia can be very useful such as in the present example where there was no anterograde conduction and analysis of retrograde conduction was obscured by excellent AV node conduction. During entrainment at a rate slightly faster than the intrinsic rate of tachycardia, the AP is activated orthodromically to the circuit and the AV node is activated both antidromically (retrograde AV node conduction) and orthodromically via the advanced atrial activation over the AP. This is verified during ablation when loss of AP conduction resulted in complete VA block for one cycle. Absence of retrograde AV node conduction after this cycle is best explained by concealed anterograde conduction in the AV node by the previous atrial activation over the AP. The ventricular cycle following the totally blocked one procedes retrogradely over the normal AV conduction system. Continuation of pacing after block over the AP allows for a stable catheter position throughout the delivery of current.

# Figure 5–10A

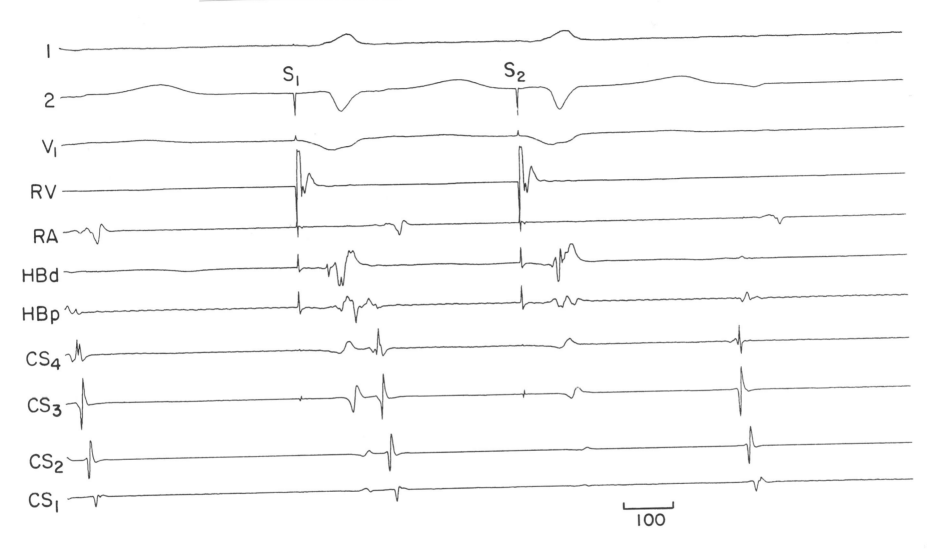

The record was obtained from a patient immediately after apparently successful ablation of a left lateral AP. $S_1$ is the last drive beat and $S_2$ is a ventricular extrastimulus. What is the observation and its significance?

## Figure 5–10B

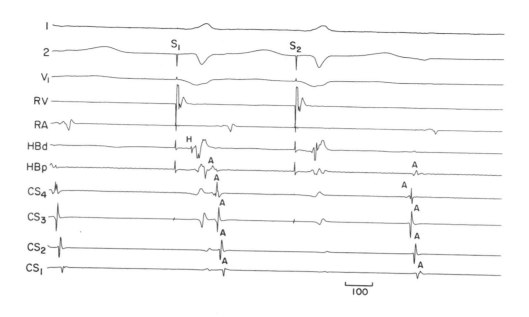

## Explanation:

Atrial activation sequence during the drive cycle is compatible with conduction over the normal AV conduction system with central atrial activation sequence clearly preceded by a His deflection. With the extrastimulus, the His appears to be displaced into the QRS, the VA conduction time prolongs considerably, and the atrial activation sequence is altered with earliest activation now in the proximal coronary sinus near the orifice ($CS_4$, $CS_3$ early). This in all probability represents conduction over a slow, posterior AV node pathway although a decremental, unidirectional posteroseptal pathway could not be definitively ruled out from this tracing. Dual AV node pathway physiology commonly coexists with the Wolff-Parkinson-White syndrome as well as the general population but ablation is only indicated if it can be related to a clinically relevant tachycardia.

## Figure 5–11A

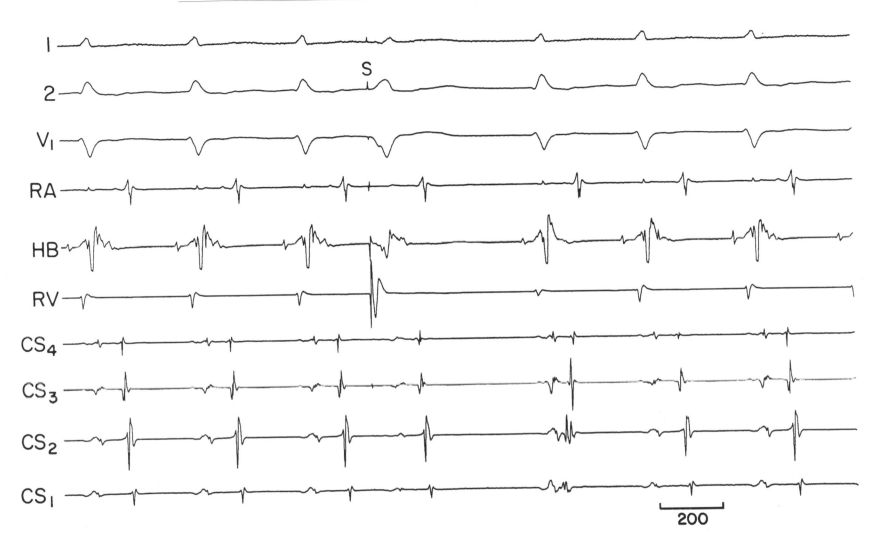

I

2
S

V₁

RA

HB

RV

CS₄

CS₃

CS₂

CS₁

200

This patient has a right anteroseptal preexcitation pattern during sinus rhythm. A PVC introduced into ongoing supraventricular tachycardia yielded the phenomena shown. What needs to be ablated?

# Figure 5–11B

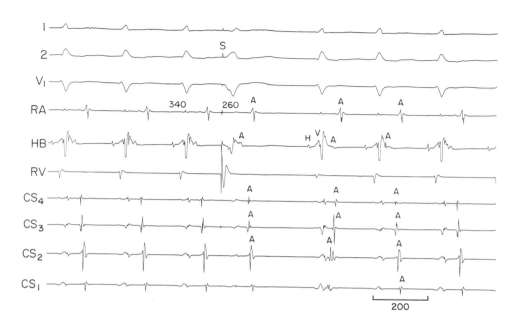

## Explanation:

The first three cycles of tachycardia represent tachycardia as was repeatedly induced in this individual and demonstrated to be AV reentry utilizing a right anteroseptal pathway as the retrograde limb. Note that earliest atrial activation is at the His site. A PVC with the stimulus artifact inscribed approximately 50 ms in front of the destined His (not seen) preexcited the atrium with no change in the activation sequence. The subsequent AH is very long and the first cycle after the PVC is associated with a different atrial preexcitation pattern, suggestive of a left lateral AP. The subsequent AH shortened and the former retrograde atrial activation pattern over the right anteroseptal pathway resumed. This patient clearly has a second left lateral AP. However, this pathway has a relatively long refractory period and is only seen after a very long AH interval. Sustained tachycardia over this pathway could not be demonstrated and, arguably, this pathway would not require ablation.

This patient also has dual AV node pathway physiology (the AV node curve relating AH to prematurity of an atrial extrastimulus was discontinuous after ablation) as evidenced by the long AH observed after the PVC during tachycardia. The slow pathway would not require ablation in its own right unless it could be demonstrated that it was capable of participating in AV node reentry. A clue that the patient does not have sustained AV node reentry is the absence of an AV node echo after the long AH. The right anteroseptal pathway is the "culprit" pathway and is the only one requiring ablation in this patient.

# *Figure 5–12A*

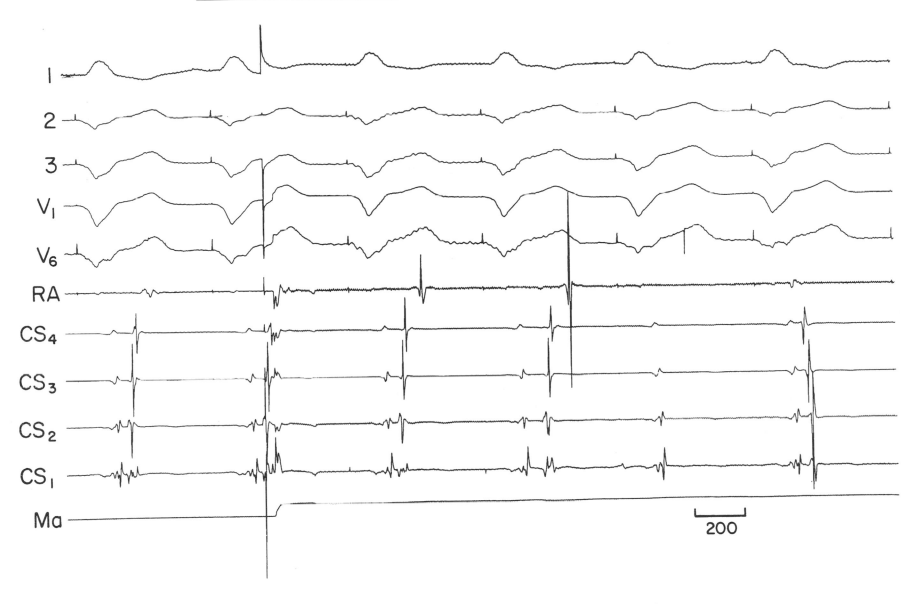

The tracing was taken from a patient undergoing ablation of a left lateral AP that was done during ventricular pacing. How many APs are involved?

# Figure 5-12B

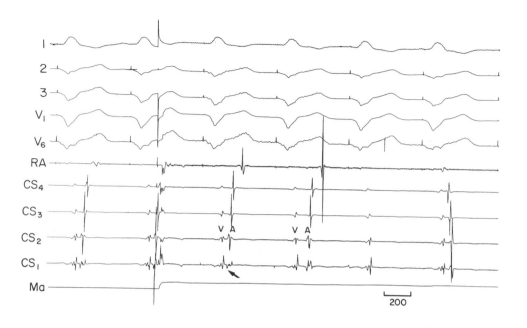

## Explanation:

Ablation was targeted by using the distal CS electrode (ablation catheter not shown). A potential (*arrow*), assumed to be an AP potential, was recorded. The retrograde atrial activation sequence shifted abruptly with the second paced cycle after the onset of current. The VA conduction time is now considerably longer with a subtle shift in activation sequence and electrogram morphology. The third cycle blocked completely and the fourth cycle was probably a sinus escape cycle (high right atrial electrogram first). It is our view that the sequence of events is best explained by two very closely spaced pathways that are both ablated at one site in the temporal sequence observed. This is suggested by the slight change in atrial activation that would not be expected to change if the injury was merely prolonging atrial conduction time. The two closely spaced pathways could be entirely distinct or interconnected (branching).

# Figure 5–13A

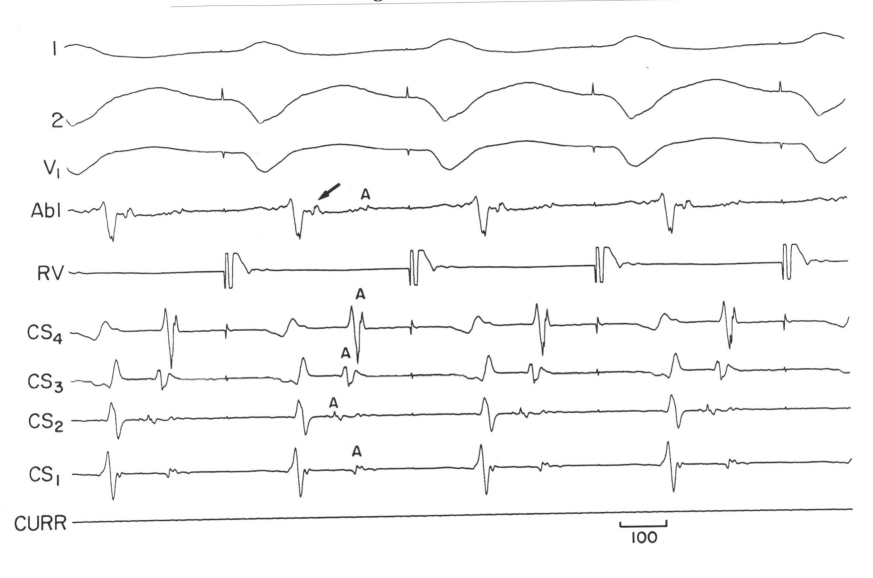

The record was taken from a patient undergoing ablation of a left lateral AP (subvalvular approach). Is this a reasonable ablation site?

# Figure 5–13B

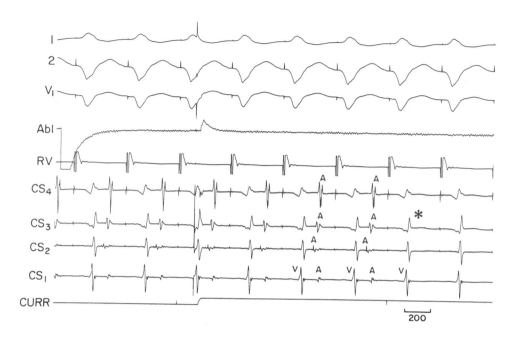

## Explanation:

The ablation catheter in this instance was directed toward the distal coronary sinus ($CS_2$) at the site of earliest atrial activation. At this site, an adequate atrial electrogram could not be recorded and the late deflection labeled as A at the ablation site was of low amplitude and arguably not even an atrial deflection. Nonetheless, a potential felt to be an AP potential (*arrow*) was observed though not validated.

In this instance, the pathway blocked after the fourth cycle after onset of current (denoted by an asterisk, *). The general teaching is that ablation of an AP at the AV ring requires both adequate atrial and ventricular deflections to indicate that it is truly at the ring. Nonetheless, the recording of a potential will allow ablation of the pathway at its ventricular insertion site even in the absence of a believable atrial electrogram.

# Figure 5-14A

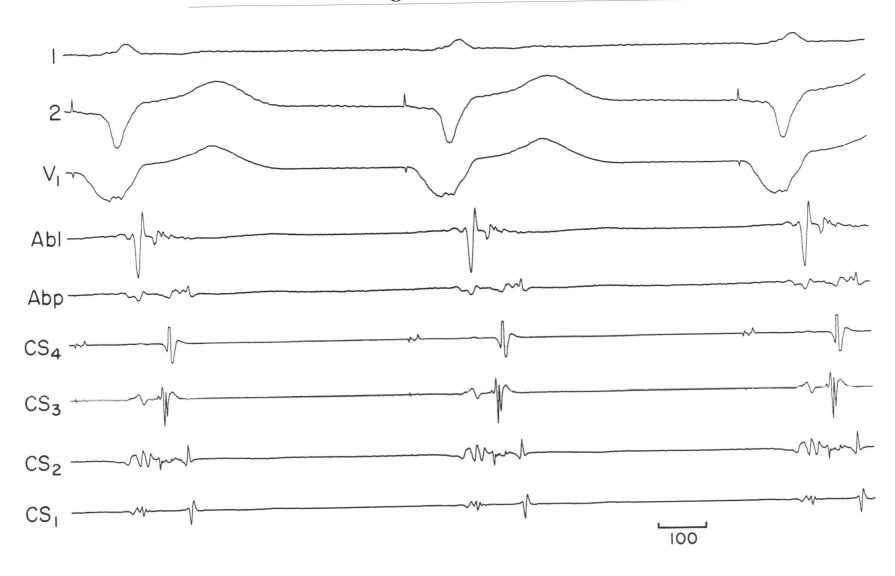

This patient was undergoing ablation of the left lateral AP. What would be a better site for ablation, $CS_3$ or $CS_2$?

# *Figure 5–14B*

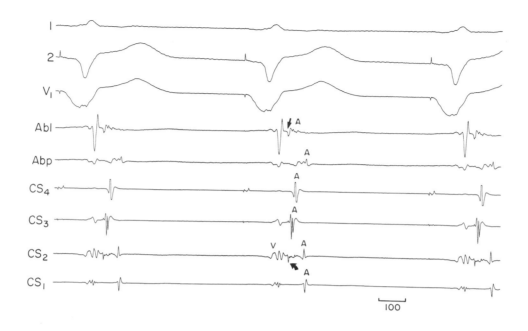

## Explanation:

Earliest retrograde atrial activation during ventricular pacing was observed posterolaterally (CS$_3$) approximately 20 mm from the CS os. However, a distinct AP potential (*lower arrow*) was observed at CS$_2$, 10 mm more distal than CS$_3$. The A deflection at CS$_2$ is much later than the earliest A. This is compatible with the ventricular insertion site recorded more distally along the CS with a pathway slanting more medially to provide atrial activation earliest at CS$_3$. The ablation catheter was positioned subvalvularly in an attempt to approximate the electrode at CS$_2$, and a similar recording showing a putative pathway potential (*upper arrow*) was seen. Ablation at this site was successful, again illustrating the value of the pathway potential in guiding ablation.

# Figure 5–15A

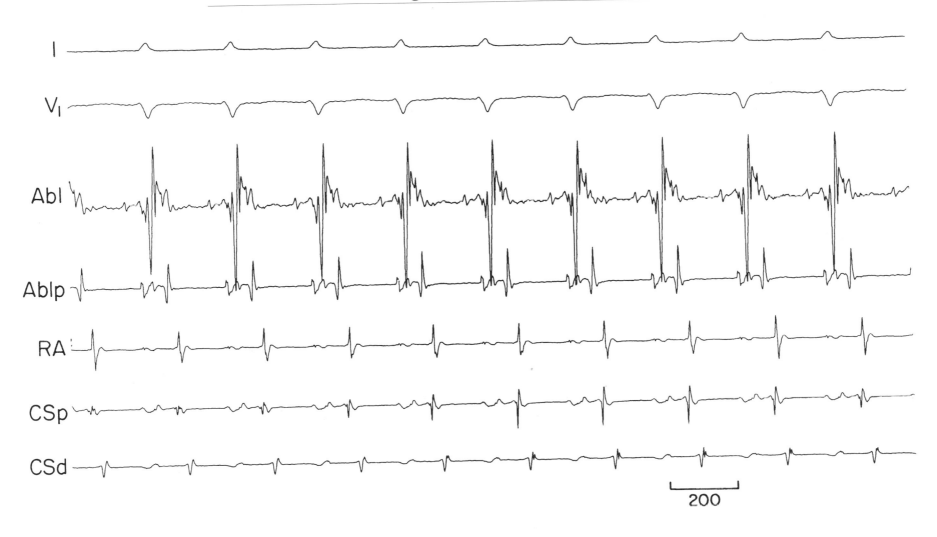

I

V$_I$

Abl

Ablp

RA

CSp

CSd

200

This patient had a right anteroseptal preexcitation pattern (same patient as Figure 5–11) and supraventricular tachycardia using a right anteroseptal pathway as the retrograde pathway. Is this a suitable ablation site?

# Figure 5–15B

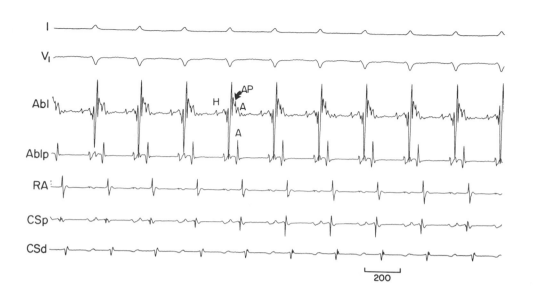

## Explanation:

By definition, the right anteroseptal AP is located in proximity to the penetrating His bundle, and both a His spike and AP potential (*arrow*) can be recorded at the same site. Ideally, the His deflection should be lower in amplitude and less rapid (more far field), whereas the pathway potential should be maximized in amplitude and slope.

This ideal ratio should be carefully sought. In this example, the labeled pathway potential has a larger amplitude and is "sharper" than the His potential. Furthermore, the atrial deflection is relatively small, supporting a more distal catheter position that would be less likely to result in AV block. Ablation during tachycardia in this instance will also allow one to monitor the AV node during ablation.

# Figure 5–16A

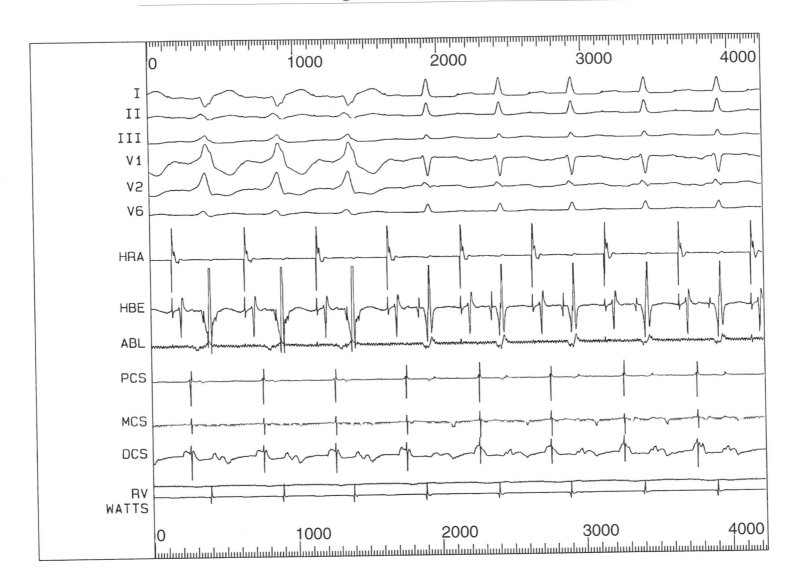

This patient was undergoing ablation of a left lateral AP. Approximately 7 s after onset of radiofrequency energy the observation shown in Fig. 5–16A was made. Is this a successful ablation?

# Figure 5-16B

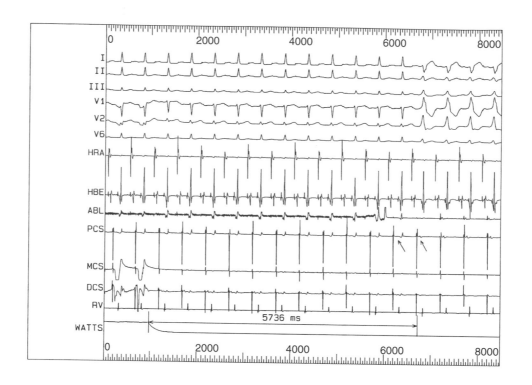

## Explanation:

This figure demonstrates that AP conduction returned approximately 6 s after radiofrequency energy was discontinued. Simultaneous tracings were recorded from the high right atrium (HRA), His bundle area (HBE), ablation catheter (ABL), proximal (PCS), mid (MCS), and distal (DCS) coronary sinus electrode, and the right ventricle (RV). The arrows point to the local AV interval on the proximal CS electrode. The last normal QRS complex has a widely spaced A and V electrogram, but when preexcitation returns the AV interval shortens due to local activation of the ventricle over the AP. Although the initial observation in Fig. 5-16A was encouraging, this merely represented the effects of increased heat to prevent AP conduction, and not destruction of the AP complex. The AP was successfully ablated with slight movement of the catheter to an adjacent area. When loss of AP conduction occurs during energy delivery, the catheter is close to the AP because the heat is transmitted only for a short distance from the catheter tip. Clearly, loss of AP conduction during energy delivery does not always represent permanent destruction of the pathway.

## *Figure 5–17A*

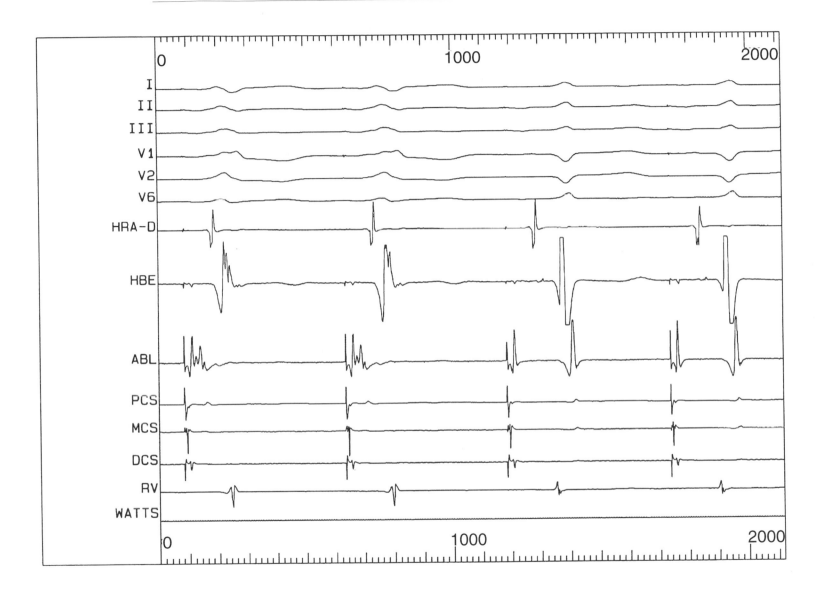

Mapping was performed prior to energy delivery in this patient with a left free wall AP.
Would you anticipate successful catheter ablation of the AP at this site?

## Figure 5–17B

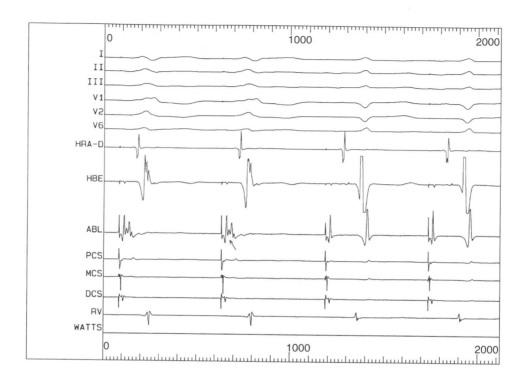

**Explanation:**

Energy delivery at this site has an extremely high chance to ablate successfully AP conduction. Note the arrow pointing to a triphasic local electrogram at the ablation site. The atrial electrogram is large, and the arrow points to a probable AP potential between the atrial and ventricular local electrograms. More important is the effect of local trauma ("bump map") to the AP, as demonstrated in the last two complexes. Loss of preexcitation occurs due to catheter pressure and the local AV interval markedly separates without the AP potential visible any longer. Ablation at this site, which was performed quickly after this observation occurred, produced permanent block over the AP. Although demonstration of an AP potential at the site of ablation is usually predictive for subsequent successful destruction of the AP with energy delivery, local trauma to the AP with catheter pressure is an even better predictor of success.

## Figure 5–18A

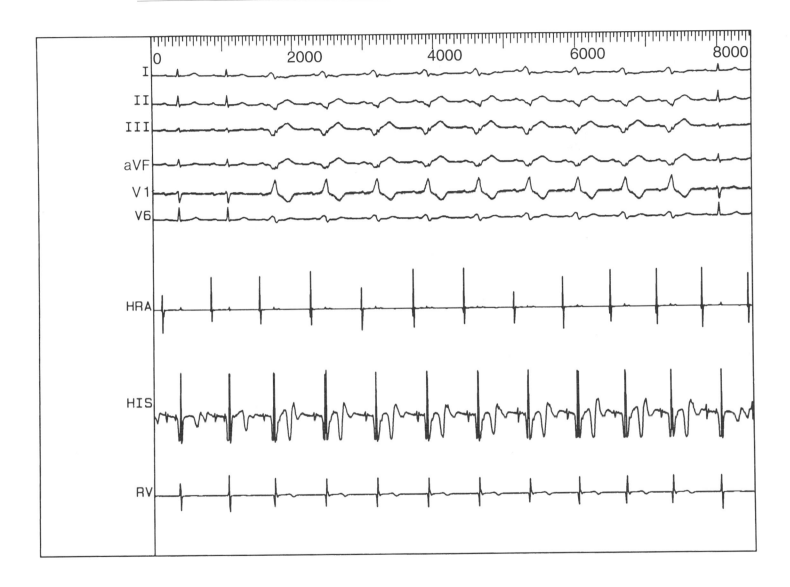

This patient has a history of documented paroxysmal SVT. No prior electrophysiologic study has been performed. Would a single catheter approach to ablate the AP likely cure this patient?

# Figure 5-18B

SVT

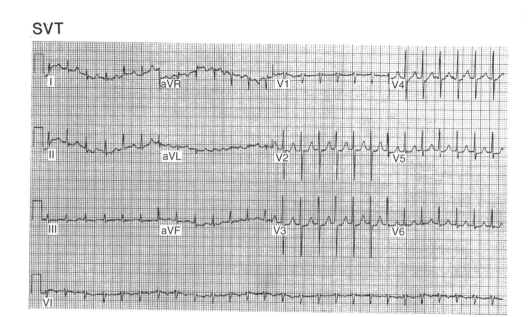

## Explanation:

This patient had an AP with intermittent anterograde conduction, but no retrograde conduction. His clinical arrhythmia was AV node reentry as seen here in the 12-lead electrocardiogram. Note the typical small $r'$ in V1 during tachycardia. Use of a single catheter ablation approach to destroy the AP would have resulted in a cosmetic alteration of the electrocardiogram without cure of this patient's tachycardia. In our opinion, it is important to document the cause of tachycardia and formulate an ablation plan based on physiologic data. Playing the odds will usually work, but we have seen a variety of arrhythmias, including VT, occur in patients with ventricular preexcitation in whom the AP does not participate in tachycardia.

# *Figure 5–19A*

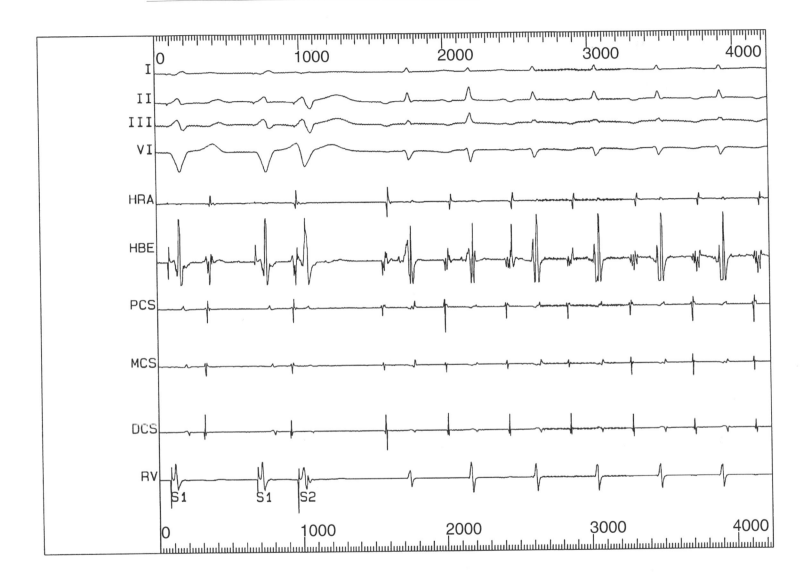

This tracing was recorded during an EP study prior to attempts at radiofrequency catheter ablation. Will ablation at a single site cure this patient?

## *Figure 5–19B*

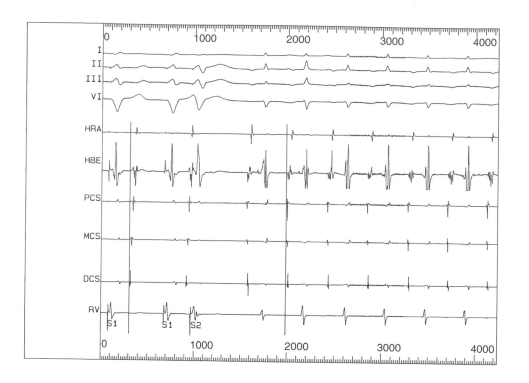

**Explanation:**

The arrhythmia induced in this tracing is a long RP tachycardia with initial atrial activation occurring near the CS os in the posteroseptal area of the right atrium. The differential diagnosis is fast/slow AV node reentry, AV reentry utilizing a slowly conducting retrograde pathway, and atrial tachycardia. Subsequent EP pacing maneuvers diagnosed AV node reentry. However, careful inspection of the initial S1 paced beat reveals a different retrograde atrial activation sequence.

This patient also had a concealed left lateral AP that could be used in AV reentry. The CS catheter was initially positioned with the proximal electrode close to the CS os, and when the catheter was advanced more laterally the eccentric atrial activation sequence became more obvious. Thus, a single catheter ablation site did not cure this patient.

# Figure 5–20A

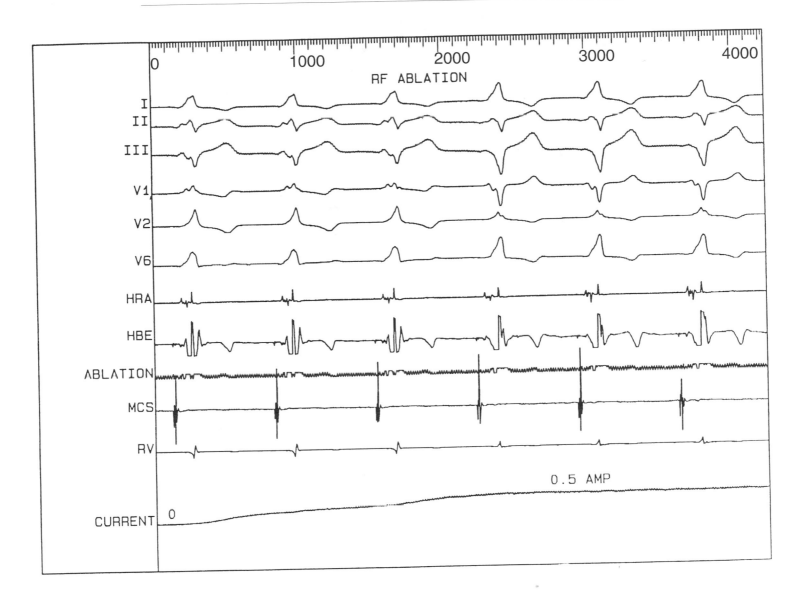

This patient was undergoing ablation of a left posterior AP. Should current application be continued?

# Figure 5–20B

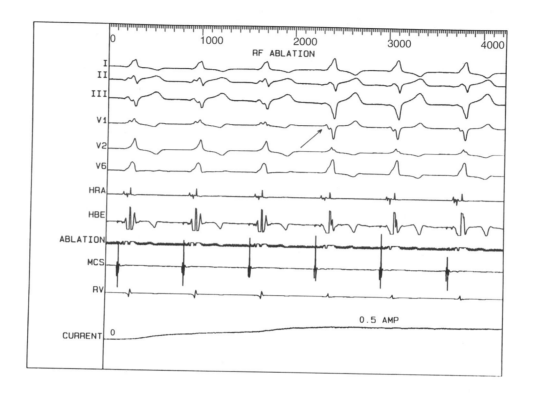

Figure 5–20B

**Explanation:**

An excellent site was selected and radiofrequency energy was initiated. Note that the fourth QRS complex has a change in morphology (*arrow*). Although preexcitation is still present, the preexcited QRS pattern has changed. The first three complexes demonstrate an upright delta wave in V1 that becomes negative in the fourth and subsequent complexes. This patient did have successful ablation of the left posterior AP, but a second AP became apparent and it was located in the right posteroseptal area. Another ablation attempt in the right posteroseptal area produced block over the second AP. Even then this patient was not cured. Tachycardia could be reinduced and complete mapping revealed a left lateral AP that had not been evident prior to ablation of the first two APs. A third ablation had to be performed, after which the patient was cured permanently.

# Figure 5-21A

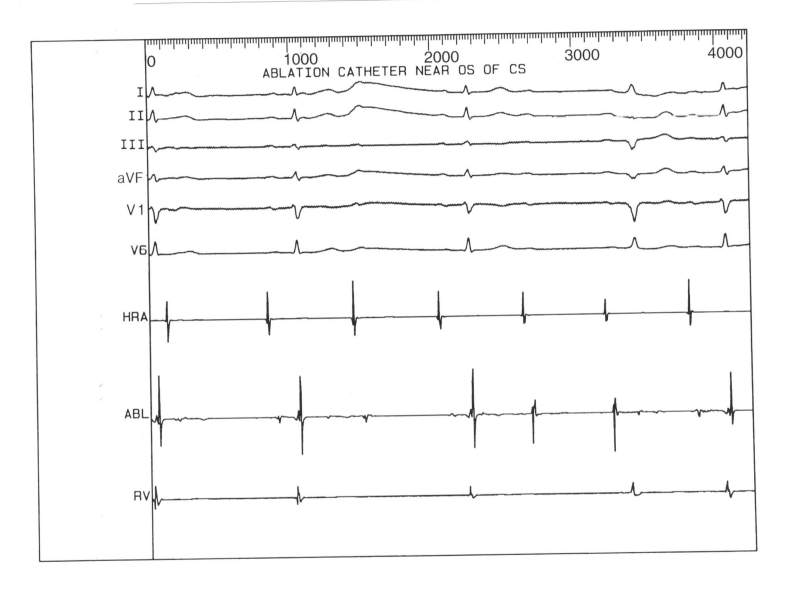

ABLATION CATHETER NEAR OS OF CS

This patient had typical slow/fast AV node reentry. The ablation catheter was positioned in the area of the CS os. Is this a good ablation site to initiate radiofrequency energy?

# Figure 5-21B

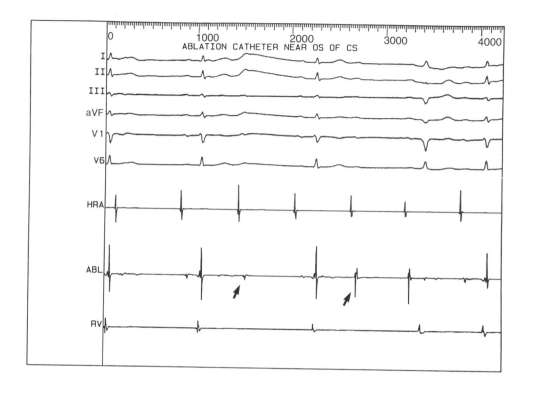

## Explanation:

It would not be wise to introduce energy at this catheter ablation site. Note that intermittent heart block occurs (*arrows*). This suggests that catheter trauma of AV nodal conduction is occurring, and another ablation site should be chosen to avoid permanent heart block with introduction of energy. There can be considerable variation in the position of the AV node in relation to the CS os. Placement of the ablation catheter near the os of the coronary sinus does not imply that one is always a "safe" distance from the AV node. When doubt exists, one can move the catheter more posteriorly. Whenever there is concern about the anatomical relationship between the ablation catheter position and AV node, energy should be introduced at relatively low levels and progressively tritrated upward.

## *Figure 5–22A*

## Site 5

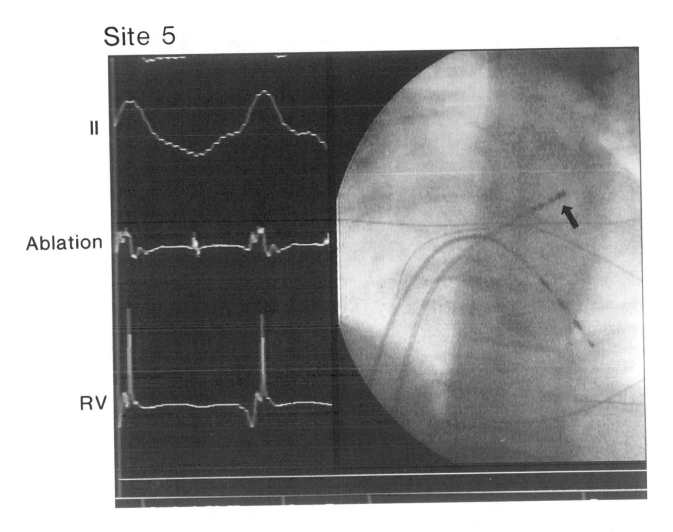

This patient had cardiomyopathy and a ventricular tachycardia occurring in the right ventricular outflow tract area. The radiograph on the right side of this figure shows the position of the ablation catheter (*arrow*) in the right ventricular outflow tract. The electrogram from the distal electrode pair is demonstrated on the left side of this figure. Is this a good site to introduce radiofrequency energy?

# Figure 5–22B

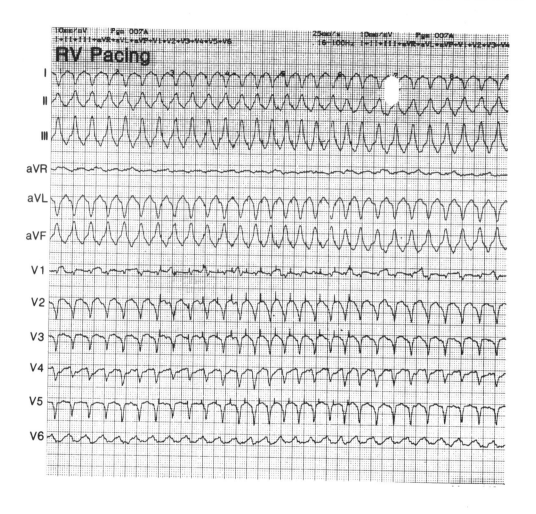

## Explanation:

The electrogram noted in Fig. 5–22A reveals a mid-diastolic potential during ventricular tachycardia. This is usually an excellent site for ablation in patients with structural heart disease. In patients with right ventricular outflow tract tachycardias and no structural heart disease, mid-diastolic potentials are not typically recorded. Figure 5–22B demonstrates paced mapping from this site. Note the excellent concordant 12-lead electrocardiogram during VT and local RV pacing. Introduction of radiofrequency energy is shown in Fig. 5–22C, and tachycardia is terminated even before full power is reached.

Figure 5–22C

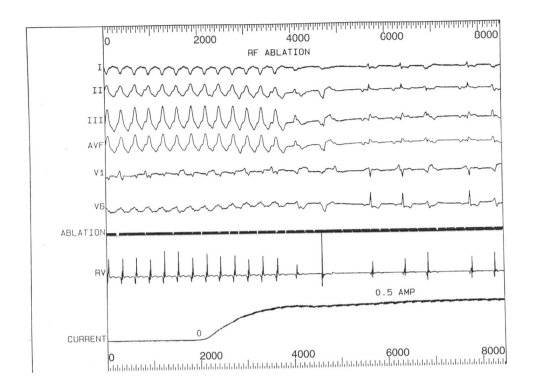

# Figure 5–23A

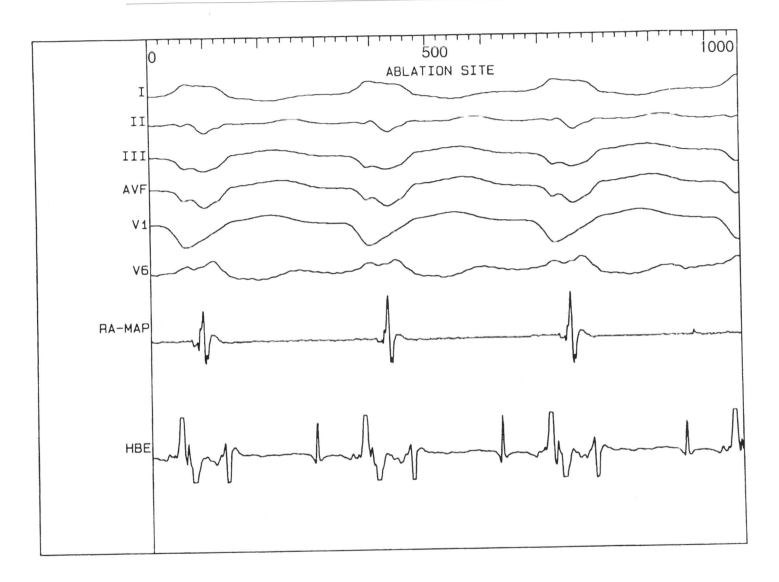

ABLATION SITE

This patient had atrial tachycardia and was undergoing mapping prior to radiofrequency ablation. Left bundle branch block aberrancy is present. Is this a good ablation site?

# Figure 5-23B

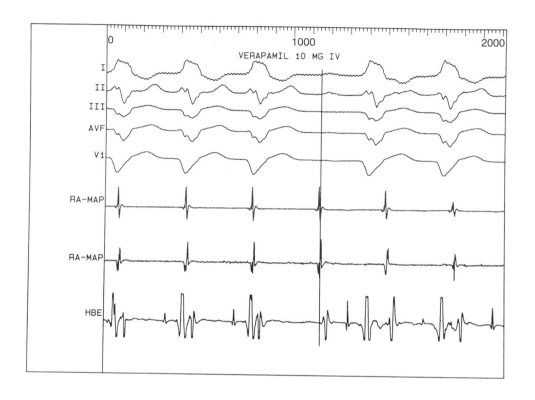

**Explanation:**

It is very difficult to know if the recorded atrial electrogram at the ablation site in Fig. 5–23A is early in relation to the surface P wave. Thus, one would try to identify the P wave prior to onset of energy delivery. There are several methods to do this. In this case verapamil was given as demonstrated in Fig. 5–23B. Atrial tachycardia continues undisturbed during AV nodal block. With block, there is a clearly defined P wave and the local atrial electrogram clearly precedes the P wave by a significant interval. An alternative method is introduction of one or more premature ventricular complexes during tachycardia to produce retrograde concealed conduction in the AV node. In this instance the P wave may become visible for one complex, and the relationship of the local atrial electrogram to the P wave can be ascertained. This patient had successful ablation of the atrial tachycardia as shown in Fig. 5–23C.

## Figure 5–23C

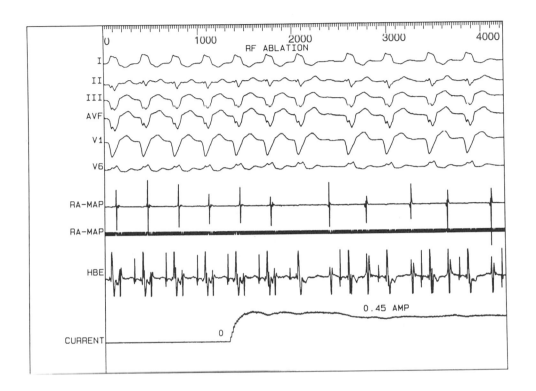

# Figure 5–24A

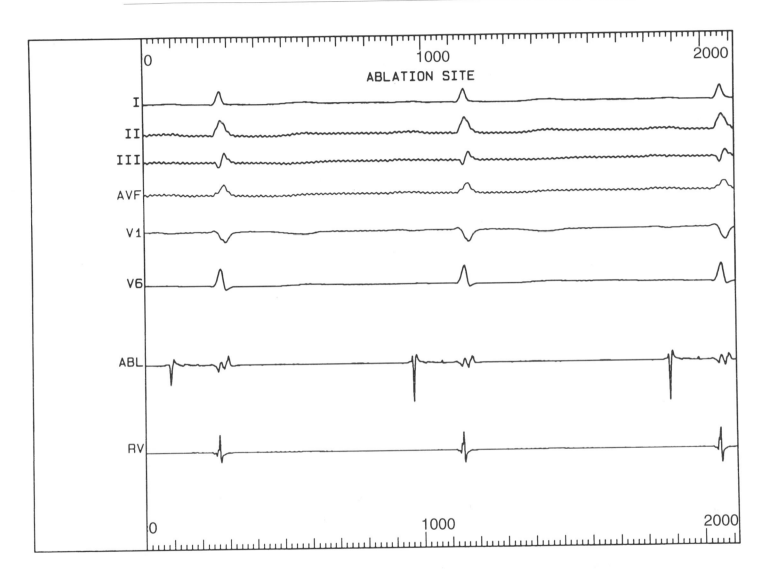

This patient had recurrent atrial fibrillation uncontrolled with multiple antiarrhythmic agents. Radiofrequency ablation of the AV junction to create complete heart block was performed. Is this a good ablation site?

# *Figure 5–24B*

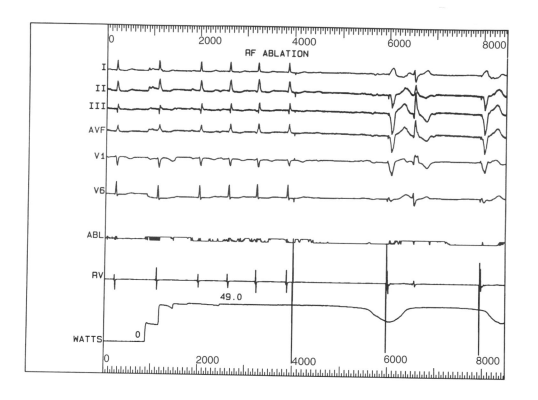

## Explanation:

Onset of radiofrequency energy at this site produced almost instantaneous rapid junctional tachycardia and complete heart block shortly thereafter. After discontinuation of energy, an electrocardiogram was recorded and is shown in Fig. 5–24C. Note that this patient has a narrow QRS escape rhythm that was stable. The ablation site in Fig. 5–24A had excellent local electrogram characteristics for AV junctional ablation. Note the large A wave with a smaller His bundle deflection. This suggests a more proximal site and after ablation the patient typically has a reasonably stable junctional escape rhythm.

A permanent pacemaker is necessary, but it is somewhat reassuring to have a backup junctional escape rhythm. Many use the term *His bundle ablation*. The His bundle is encased in the central fibrous body and is very difficult to destroy with usual radiofrequency energy catheter systems. It is much more likely that the AV node is damaged in most patients. However, the more distal the ablation site, the less likely a stable narrow QRS junctional rhythm will be present after ablation.

## After AVJ Ablation

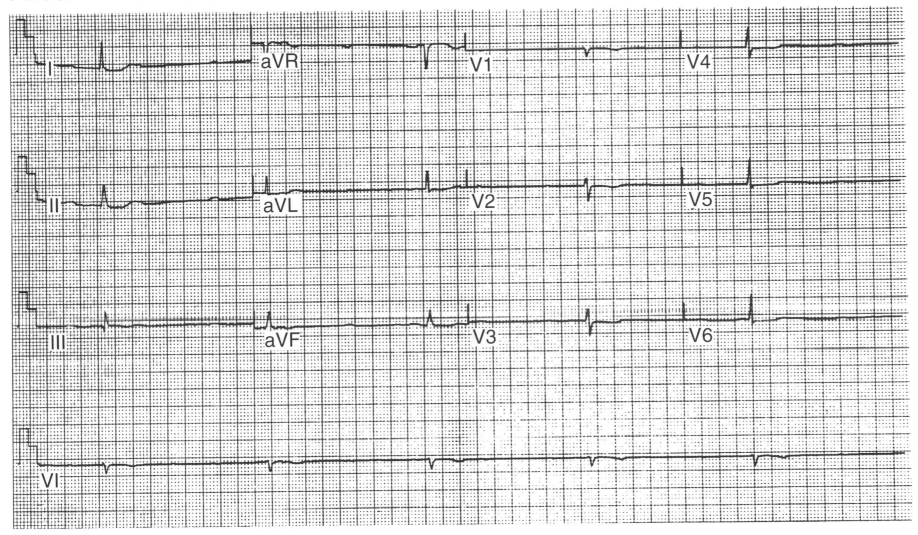

# Figure 5–25A

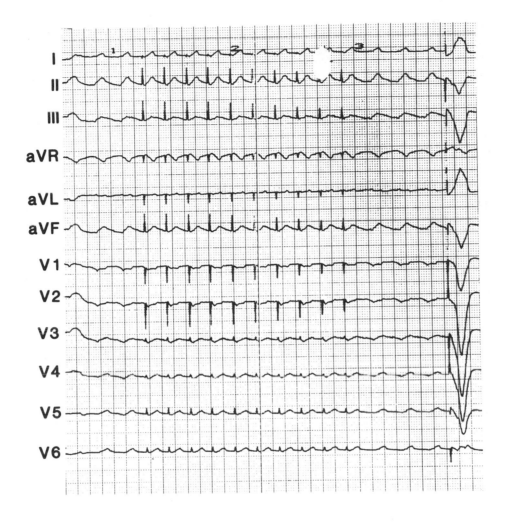

This patient had persistent atrial flutter unresponsive to multiple antiarrhythmic drugs. Radiofrequency ablation was performed to cure the atrial flutter. The patient also had extremely poor AV node conduction and had a permanent dual chamber pacemaker in place.

Prior to introduction of radiofrequency energy, pacing was performed at the ablation site. Does this appear to be a good site for ablation?

## *Figure 5–25B*

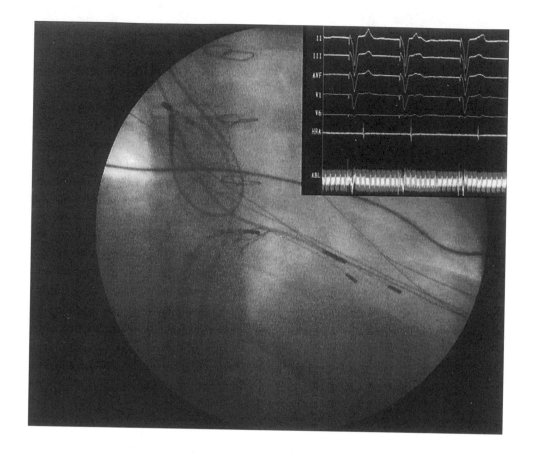

### Explanation:

The ablation catheter was positioned in an area posterior to the CS os in the AV groove as noted in Fig. 5–25B. In Fig. 5–25A, pacing entrains the P waves during atrial flutter and the morphology of the paced and spontaneous P waves is nearly identical. Thus, the catheter must be very close to or within the tachycardia circuit. The stimulus to P wave is rather short, suggesting the catheter position is near the exit point in the isthmus of slow conduction in the circuit. Onset of radiofrequency energy at this site resulted in termination of atrial flutter (Fig. 5–25C), and flutter has not recurred in this patient during long-term follow-up.

It is useful to verify conduction block in the isthmus after RF ablation. This can be done by analyzing the conduction pattern and time from a pacing site near the CS os to the low lateral right atrium.

## *Figure 5–25C*

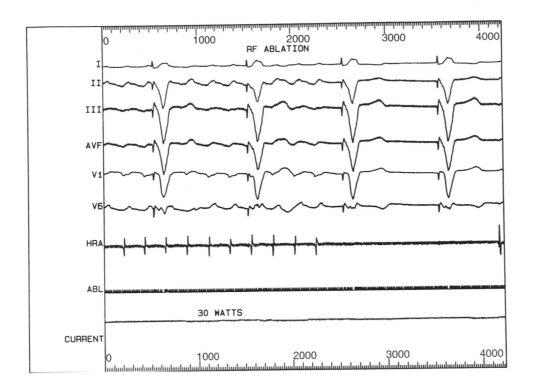

# Index

# *Index*

ISBN 0-07-035169-4

EAN

9 780070 351691

90000>

KLEIN/PRYSTOW CLIN ELEC RE